D1783931

# Contents

# List of tables

# A POCKETBOOK OF

# Palliative Care

## ROBIN HULL
MB, BS, FRCGP

*Prefessor of General Practice*
*Free University of Amsterdam*

*Macmillian Senior Lecturer*
*in*
*Palliative Care*
*Birmingham University*
*Medical School*

**McGRAW-HILL BOOK COMPANY Sydney**
New York  San Francisco  Auckland  Bogotá
Caracas  Lisbon  London  Madrid  Mexico City
Milan  Montreal  New Delhi  San Juan
Singapore  Tokyo  Toronto

*For Gillian,*

*who knows about pain,*

*with love.*

**National Library of Australia Cataloguing-in-Publication data:**

Hull, Robin.
  A pocketbook of palliative care.

  Bibliography.
  Includes index.
  ISBN 0 07 470138 X.

  1. Palliative treatment – Handbooks, manuals, etc. I. Title.

362.175

Published in Australia by
**McGraw-Hill Book Company Australia Pty Limited**
**4 Barcoo Street, Roseville NSW 2069, Australia**
Typeset in Australia by Craftsmen Type & Art
Printed in Australia by Star Printery Pty Ltd
Sponsoring Editor John Rowe
Production Editors Marjorie Pressley and Diana Hill
Designer George Sirrett (Asymmetric Typography Pty Ltd)

# Preface

Many people have influenced this book. It began as a request from a colleague, Dr Martin Kendall at Birmingham Medical School, that I write a series of articles for the *Journal of Clinical Pharmacy and Therapeutics*[1-7] published by Blackwell Scientific Publications of Oxford. Though it is designed to slip into the white coat pocket of the newly qualified house officer or the bag of a trainee general practitioner it is also a useful introduction to palliative care for medical students and nurses.

The book is based mainly on hospice care in England but I have also drawn on experience in North America and Australia. It includes information about the treatment of the commoner problems of the care of patients with advanced cancer or AIDS with both conventional and complementary treatment. It also offers help and advice on supporting the dying and on that most difficult of all human tasks, the breaking of bad news. Finally it describes how additional help may be obtained for patients with cancer either from hospices or from a multitude of helping agencies and support groups throughout the world.

## Acknowledgments

My students and patients have taught me so much about caring for people with cancer and AIDS that they need first acknowledgment. Among many who have inspired me to learn more about palliative care I must mention Balfour Mount of Montreal and Robert Twycross of Oxford. I am also indebted to Harry van Bommel and Alison Davies of Canada, Lesley Rowe of Sydney and Christine Benson of Melbourne, who helped with addresses of helping agencies in North America and Australasia. Lesley Rowe also read the manuscript, making many encouraging and helpful additions.

Lastly I am indebted to Blackwell Scientific Publications Ltd for permission to use material published in the *Journal of Clinical Pharmacy and Therapeutics* and to the editor of *Update* for material in Table 9.1.

## Publishers' note

Medicine is an ever-changing science. As new research and clinical experience broaden our knowledge, changes in treatment and drug therapy are required. The editors and the publisher of this work have checked with sources believed to be reliable in their efforts to provide information that is complete and generally in accord with the standards accepted at the time of publication. However, in view of the possibility of human error or changes in medical sciences, neither the editors, nor the publisher, nor any other party who has been involved in the preparation or publication of this work warrants that the information contained herein is in every respect accurate or complete and they are not responsible for any errors or omissions or for the results obtained from use of such information. Readers are encouraged to confirm the information contained herein with other sources. For example and in particular, readers are advised to check the product information sheet included in the package of each drug they plan to administer to be certain that the information contained in this book is accurate and that changes have not been made in the recommended dose or in the contraindications for administration. This recommendation is of particular importance in connection with new or infrequently used drugs.

## CHAPTER 1

# Introduction

CANCER is a complex concept consisting of many different diseases of differing seriousness and symptomatology. It is surrounded by a dense cloud of mythology, folk belief and superstition. A young patient dying of melanomatosis remarked to a group of my students: 'The fear of cancer is worse than cancer.' This remark underlines the importance of good communication to allay the patient's fear, which is so often based on ignorance about cancer. This is vital since listening carefully to the patient, explaining and reassuring are as important as any medication in resolving many symptoms.

Ideal palliative care depends on the twin concepts of good communication and as near perfect control of symptoms as is possible. Such control depends on accurate diagnosis followed by the application of rational therapy. The pathological nature of the patient's cancer is often irrelevant in diagnosing the cause of symptoms, except where sites of metastases or particular metabolic upsets occur in association with specific tumours. The first question must always be what is the mechanism causing this particular symptom? Since a patient may have several symptoms, even several pains, at a single time, this question needs to be asked of each symptom in turn.

When a person has metastatic cancer the first need is for expert nursing care, with attention to bowel function, pressure areas, the hundred little symptoms and the many, and often major, physical, emotional, spiritual and social problems of severe illness. The second need is for an understanding doctor, skilled in communication and in symptom control. Palliative care reaches its best when nursing and medical skills are combined. Sometimes the doctor may lead this team, quite as often it will be the nurse, but it may also be the lay carer, most often the spouse, and at times it may be the patient himself or herself. The essential requirement of good teamwork in palliative care is communication; each member of the team must be prepared to listen to and consider the suggestions of individuals from other backgrounds and skills. Though traditionally in other fields of care it may be the doctor who decides and others who carry out instructions, in good palliative care it may be the doctor's role to listen and acquiesce in the advice of nurses, clergy, social workers, the patient or the relatives. This change in role is not always easily accepted, but when the doctor does not hear then the patient may suffer.

The task of cancer care can be summed up by the fifteenth century French folk-saying:

> To cure sometimes
> To relieve often
> To comfort always

Palliation is part of cancer care and as important as prevention, diagnosis, management and terminal care, all of which are different from palliative care. Palliative care is defined as that care provided for patients in whom, after exact diagnosis, attempts to cure have been considered and abandoned. It follows that palliative care aims at increasing the patient's physical, emotional, social and spiritual quality of life. This is holism in the Smutsian sense rather than, as it has come to be, a synonym for alternative medicine (not that that has no place in palliative care). Terminal care, sometimes spoken of synonymously with palliative care, concerns the management of death itself and, though it may be part of palliative care, is distinct from it. Palliative care may be required for years, even decades, while terminal care is agonal, lasting only hours or days.

A very useful way of judging the appropriateness of any intervention is provided by Dr Balfour Mount, palliative care specialist at Montreal's Royal Victoria Hospital (personal communication):

There are only three admissible aims of treatment:
1. to cure disease;
2. to prolong life;
3. to increase the quality of life.

*All interventions should be tried against these aims; if a treatment does not satisfy at least one of these criteria then it should be abandoned.*

This short book looks at some of the problems of the care of people with advanced cancer from a symptomatic point of view. In each case, although stress is laid on diagnosis and the pharmacological basis of relief of symptoms, the importance of time to talk and listen must always be remembered.

*Note*

For Australian readers, drugs or treatments listed that are not used or are not available in Australia are indicated throughout the text by a dagger (†).

# The management of pain in advanced cancer

Pain is a complex sensation and difficult to define. Perhaps the most satisfactory working definition is from Twycross: 'that which the patient says hurts.' 'Pain is *always* physical but is *always* modified by the psyche.' (Balfour Mount)[2] Although 85–90% of cancer pain has been capable of relief by methods described by Cecily Saunders over 30 years ago, pain relief in cancer is still unacceptably bad because we do not use available treatment. Pain is an inadequate word to describe the suffering caused by advanced cancer, which may be complicated by psychological, social or spiritual factors. These non-physical aspects of pain require understanding and discussion. Patients admitted to hospices in severe pain frequently settle well with no more than a change of environment, peace and good counsel.

There may be physical pain of many different qualities and quantities. There are also preventable pains such as hunger, constipation, and mouth problems. Any or all of these may be expressed as pain and thresholds vary between individuals, influenced by physical factors such as heat or cold, or modified by emotions. Perhaps anguish* is the better, more embracing, word to describe this complicated condition.

Contrary to general opinion cancer is not painful of itself. If only it were it would not be half the problem since it would declare itself early. It is important to realise that it is what cancer does to a patient that causes pain. This means that the way in which a cancer produces pain needs exact understanding if it is to be relieved.

Physical pain occurs in about two-thirds of cancer patients, varying from 80–85% in cancers affecting bone or the cervix to 20% in lymphoma or 5% in leukaemia. Pain may be caused by many factors as listed in Table 2.1. Each of these causes of pain will need precise diagnosis of the mechanism of the pain so that the most appropriate measures for its relief may be adopted. From the list of possible causes (Table 2.1) it can be seen that pain relief in cancer may depend on the use of many drugs not normally indicated as analgesics, including: antibiotics, anticonvulsants, antidepressants, anti-inflammatory, antirheumatic, anxiolytic, spasmolytic as well as conventional analgesic drugs. Table 2.2 lists some indications of pain and their appropriate management.

Contrary to commonly held opinion opioids are not a universal panacea; some pain that will not improve with morphine will respond to other drugs. There are three sorts of pain that do not respond well to opioids: neuropathic pain, incident pain (due to positional problems, renal calculus, spinal fractures etc.) and pain with a large psychosocial component.

It is a safe rule to start with the simplest drug appropriate to the cause of pain at low dose and then to increase dose and relative analgesic potency of the drug until relief is obtained.

The drug ladder consists of:

Non-narcotic drugs → weak narcotics → strong narcotic

---

* This word derives, as does the more familiar 'angina', from the Old French *angoisse*, which meant choking. Interestingly, modern slang usage employs the word 'choked' to express extreme distress of emotional or physical form.

**Table 2.1** *Causes of pain*

1. *Tissue destruction* releases prostaglandins, histamine and bradykinins and is particularly common with bone metastases.
2. *Pressure* may occur through expansion of a tumour in a confined space.
3. *Trauma* (as in pathological fracture) is painful in itself and also because of the release of prostaglandins following tissue damage.
4. *Neurological pain* may occur from direct tumour involvement, for example in brachialgia, but may also occur as part of a generalised neuropathy associated with malignancy or because of brain involvement. Dysaesthetic nerve pain, similar to that of post herpetic neuralgia, gives rise to superficial burning pain.
5. Pain may also arise because of *muscle spasm*, particularly in the back and shoulders, where it is often related to anxiety or stress.
6. Secondary *infection* may be a cause of pain, particularly in the head and neck, in pelvic cancers or in fungating breast lesions.
7. *Ischaemic pain* may arise because a tumour has outgrown its blood supply or is occluding blood vessels.
8. *Tenesmoid pain*, due to smooth muscle spasm, may occur in rectal cancers.
9. *Disturbed metabolism* may exacerbate existing pain in hypercalcaemia and uraemia or give rise to intense pruritus in obstructive jaundice.
10. It is also important to remember that patients may have multiple pathology and that pain may be related to other conditions such as arthritis.

---

A patient may have several different pains at once, each requiring separate diagnosis and appropriate management, not necessarily involving the use of drugs. In the presence of severe pain lesser pains may not be noticed but may become apparent once the severe pain is controlled. Where the pain is thought to arise from tissue destruction, for example in the presence of bone metastases, antiprostaglandin drugs such as aspirin or a non-steroidal anti-inflammatory drug (NSAID) will be the drug of choice. Pressure may cause pain where a tumour is expanding within a closed space as in subperiosteal or intracranial lesions. In such cases the reduction of tumour bulk by surgery, radiotherapy or steroids may be the best way of relieving pain.

Table 2.2 *Drugs used in treatment of pain*

| Indication | Drug | Route | Dose |
|---|---|---|---|
| Tissue destruction NSAIDs | Aspirin | Oral | 300–900 4 hourly |
| | Ibuprofen | Oral | 1.2–1.6 g/day |
| | Indomethacin | Oral | 50–200 mg/day |
| | | p.r. | 100 mg at night |
| | Naproxen | Oral | 0.5–1g/day |
| | | p.r. | 500 mg at night |
| Pressure | Dexamethasone | Oral/s.c. | 2–16 mg/day |
| Neurological pain | Amitriptyline | Oral | 25–75 mg twice daily |
| | Carbamazepine | Oral | 100–200 mg thrice daily |
| | Sodium valproate | Oral | 0.62.5 g/day |
| Muscle spasm | Diazepam | Oral/i.v./p.r. | 2–10 mg three to four times daily |
| Tenesmus | Chlorpromazine | Oral/i.m. | 25–50 mg three to four times daily |
| Non-narcotics | Aspirin | Oral | 300–900 4 hourly |
| | Paracetamol | Oral | 0.5–1 g 4 hourly |
| Weak narcotics | Codeine | Oral | 30–60 mg 4 hourly |
| | Dextro-propoxephene[a] | Oral | 60 mg two to four times daily |
| Strong narcotics | Buprenorphine s.l. | | 200–400 µg three to four times daily |
| | Dextromoramide | Oral/s.c./p.r. | 5–20 mg p.r.n. for acute episodes of pain |
| | Diamorphine | Oral/s.c. | 2.5 mg—enough[b] 4 hourly or continuously |
| | Morphine | Oral/s.c. | 2.5 mg—enough[b] 4 hourly or continuously |

[a] Dextropropoxephene is often combined with non-narcotics (e.g. Doloxene Co, Co-Proxamol).

[b] The correct dose of opioid is that which is enough to relieve the patient's pain; it may be many grams per day.

Trauma may respond to immobilisation or, where it is due to pathological fracture, to surgical fixation, radiotherapy, NSAIDs or steroids.

Neurological pain may be due to pressure effects, direct nerve involvement, or to a generalised neuropathy. Pain may be burning or stabbing in nature (as in postherpetic neuralgia) — called dysaesthetic pain. This type of neurological pain often responds well to antidepressants such as amitriptyline. Root pain such as sciatica, brachialgia or intercostalgia will often be eased with anticonvulsants such as carbamazepine or sodium valproate. The general peripheral neuropathy of carcinomatosis is more difficult but may respond to steroids, or possibly B vitamins. There are four usual approaches to neurological pain:

- The standard approach with oral narcotics, NSAIDs and adjuvant analgesia.
- Steroids with phenytoin or carbamazepine and amitriptyline.
- Intravenous narcotics.
- Epidural narcotics.

All these help but none is the complete answer. Balfour Mount[1] recommends mexiletine, which he described as the most 'significant advance in palliative care since Cecily Saunders'. Mexiletine is an antiarrhythmic related to local anaesthetics such as procainamide. Dejgard[3] of Copenhagen reported in 1988 on pain relief in diabetic neuropathy with mexiletine, which is thought to work by blocking sodium channels. It was never very successful as a cardiac drug because of many side-effects (especially nausea and vomiting) and many CNS effects (including ataxia, ocular disturbances, convulsions) all of which were commonest when initiating intravenous therapy. It is contraindicated in hypersensitivity, heart block, with β-blockers or other antiarrhythmics, and in depressed liver function. Response is usually within days but may take some weeks. Balfour Mount[2] used it in Canada in ten patients with severe neuropathic pain, with complete relief in three, significant relief in three, some relief in three and no relief in only one.

The pain of muscle spasm may be effectively relieved by warmth, massage and anxiolytic and antispasmodic drugs such as diazepam.

Infection may cause pain by inflammation of the tumour itself or of adjacent structures such as the bladder or pleura and may require appropriate antibiotics. The pain, discomfort and the odour of infected fungating lesions may be improved with local applications of Betadine or of metronidazole gel. The pain of ischaemia may require tumour debulking by means of surgery or radiotherapy but where this is not indicated dexamethasone may be beneficial. Where pain is exacerbated by disturbed metabolic function, as in hypercalcaemia or jaundice, efforts should be made to correct this (*vide infra*).

## Opioids

Where pain is not controlled by the measures outlined above or by weak narcotic drugs such as codeine or dextropropoxyphene, then progression to opioid drugs is indicated. Morphine and diamorphine are the most important. Pethidine has no place in palliative care because of its short half-life, which provides analgesia for only 2–3 hours. In addition, pethidine in large dosage leads to accumulation of toxic metabolites. Pentazocine (Fortral) and buprenorphine (Temgesic) are not recommended in the pain control of advanced cancer because they are partial morphine antagonists. Buprenorphine is absorbed through the buccal mucosa and, because of its ease of administration, is widely used, but it may reduce the analgesia provided by morphine. Dextromoramide (Palfium) has a short duration of action and is useful as a booster analgesic before painful procedures such as changing dressings. There is little difference between diamorphine and morphine apart from a far greater solubility of the former and a slightly greater potency. Diamorphine is extremely soluble, permitting large doses to be administered in a 10 mL syringe driver. The potency of diamorphine to morphine by mouth is in the ratio of 3:2 and by injection 4:2 or 5:2. Diamorphine, which is not available in Australia or the United States, is a semisynthetic derivative of morphine and is rapidly metabolised to morphine.

**Table 2.3** *Conversion from oral morphine/diamorphine to syringe driver*

| Dosage | 4 hourly oral morphine | 4 hourly oral diamorphine | 4 hourly i.m./s.c. diamorphine injection | 24 hourly s.c. diamorphine injection |
|---|---|---|---|---|
| Starting dose (mg) | 5–10 | 2.5–7.5 | 2.5–5 | 15–30 |
| | 15 | 10 | 5 | 30 |
| | 20 | 15 | 7.5 | 45 |
| | 45 | 30 | 15 | 90 |
| Increase dose by | 60 | 40 | 20 | 120 |
| 30–50% at each | 75 | 50 | 25 | 150 |
| step | 90 | 60 | 30 | 180 |
| | 120 | 80 | 40 | 240 |
| | 300 | 200 | 100 | 600 |
| | 900 | 600 | 300 | 1800 |
| | 3000 | 2000 | 1000 | 6000 |

Dosage should be increased until pain relief is achieved without undue sedation. There appears to be no upper dose ceiling. (The largest amount I know of was 24 g of diamorphine by syringe driver in 24 hours.)

Continuous subcutaneous infusion of opioids by syringe driver is often very successful in the control of pain when drugs cannot be taken by mouth. However, it is a mistake to use this method of delivery when the oral route is possible. In Britain diamorphine is available in 100 and 500 mg ampoules in addition to the more usual smaller doses of 10 and 30 mg. When using 500 mg of diamorphine a minimum of 2 mL of water for injection should be used. Table 2.3 indicates how to convert an oral dosage to a 24 hour subcutaneous infusion dosage.

*Rules for the prescription of morphine*

1. Always prescribe the simplest route and the simplest formulation, that is, by mouth as a simple aqueous mixture of morphine sulfate.
2. Morphine produces analgesia lasting for 3–5 hours and must be given by the clock every 4 hours, **never** as required.

3. A patient's pain should be titrated with oral morphine mixture until the appropriate analgesic dose is determined, it may then be appropriate to give other forms of morphine (e.g MST Continus in UK, MS Contin in Australia).

4. MST produce analgesia lasting 12 hours provided they are swallowed whole. In most cases (98%) MST provide sustained analgesia for a full 12 hours. In a minority of cases it may be necessary to increase the frequency to three times a day. Pain is always easier to prevent than to treat when it is present.

It must always be remembered that *in the presence of severe pain* morphine:

- in correct dosage does **not** depress respiration;
- does **not** cause addiction;
- may induce vomiting initially, but this is **not** a problem of continued use;
- *always causes constipation, so concurrent prescription of aperients is essential.*

*An important point about respiratory depression*: if pain is relieved (e.g. by nerve blockade in a patient receiving high-dose morphine) then respiratory embarrassment may follow. It is therefore important to reduce morphine following such procedures. Failure to do this may require administration of naloxone to protect against respiratory depression.

## Other forms of pain relief

*For pain of increased intracranial pressure*
In severe headache associated with raised intracranial pressure there is evidence that very high doses of steroids may be helpful and produce immediate effect. It is not known why, but their action is clearly too fast to be due to reduction of peritumoural oedema. It has been suggested that relief may be related to a vascular

component in the pain. Pain relief also lasts for many hours. Balfour Mount described a case of cerebral tumour in which the patient appeared to be dying and in very severe pain. He gave intravenous dexamethasone with immediate relief of pain. The patient did not die and the pain returned so the dexamethasone was repeated for several weeks at dosages varying from 60 mg bd to 40 mg tid. Eventually the dose was reduced to a maintenance of 20 mg tid, which kept the patient pain free until his death several weeks later. In a photograph taken just before his death, the patient looked comparatively normal without the gross Cushingism one might expect. Side-effects of dexamethasone appear to be very much less marked when used intravenously.

*Radiotherapy*

Radiotherapy is a potent pain reliever particularly where pain is caused by bony metastases. The presence of spinal pain should always alert the carer to the possibility of the preventable emergency of paraplegia, which may be avoided with early radiotherapy.

*Nerve blockade*

It may sometimes be necessary to destroy pain pathways by nerve block. These techniques are difficult and require the expertise of experienced anaesthetists to block dorsal roots, the coeliac or brachial plexus. When all else has failed division of the spinothalamic tract of the spinal cord may be considered. Where pain is relieved after surgical blockade it is important to reduce the dose of opioids (*vide supra*).

Non-destructive pain relief can sometimes be dramatically achieved with transcutaneous nerve stimulation (TENS). Methods employed by practitioners of alternative medicine should not be ruled out; if the patient derives benefit the treatment is worthwhile however bizarre it may seem.

# Summarising the management of pain

1. Take a careful history exploring all aspects of pain: physical, psychological, social and spiritual. This alone will help enormously since patients need to feel that their pain is understood and appreciated.
2. Identify each of the several different pains a patient is aware of.
3. Explore the causation of each pain separately and treat appropriately.
4. Use coanalgesia before starting strong analgesics.
5. Where opioids are required titrate the dose, reassuring the patient that adequate pain control will be forthcoming once the correct dose is determined.
6. When the appropriate dosage is determined change to long-acting opioid preparations (MST or MS Contin).
7. Review continuously, being prepared to change drug or dose.
8. When making changes only make one alteration at a time since it is not possible to know which of several changes has produced good (or bad) effect.
9. Remember that the best analgesic is often the close attention to detail provided by a visibly interested and caring doctor or nurse.

## CHAPTER 3

# Gastrointestinal symptoms

## Nausea and vomiting

Nausea and vomiting occur in about one-third of patients with advanced cancer and rational management depends on precise diagnosis of cause. The vomiting centre and the chemoreceptor trigger zone lying in the floor of the fourth ventricle respond to a variety of stimuli by inducing nausea or vomiting. The causes of nausea and vomiting are shown in Figure 3.1. Nausea and vomiting may be induced by any combination of six main causes:

- psychological factors;
- vestibular disturbance;
- toxic effects due to drugs or abnormal metabolites;
- factors within the gastrointestinal tract (constipation, obstruction etc.);
- raised intracranial pressure;
- environmental factors such as discomfort, heat and strong odours.

The mechanism of induction of vomiting is controlled by the inter-reaction of the vestibular apparatus, the vomiting centre and the chemoreceptor zone (see Fig. 3.1). Both the vestibular apparatus and the vomiting centre have acetylcholine and histamine ($H_1$) receptors and nausea caused by the effects of these substances is likely to respond to treatment with antihistamines or anticholinergics. The chemoreceptor zone has dopamine ($D_2$) receptors. Nausea caused by factors influencing the

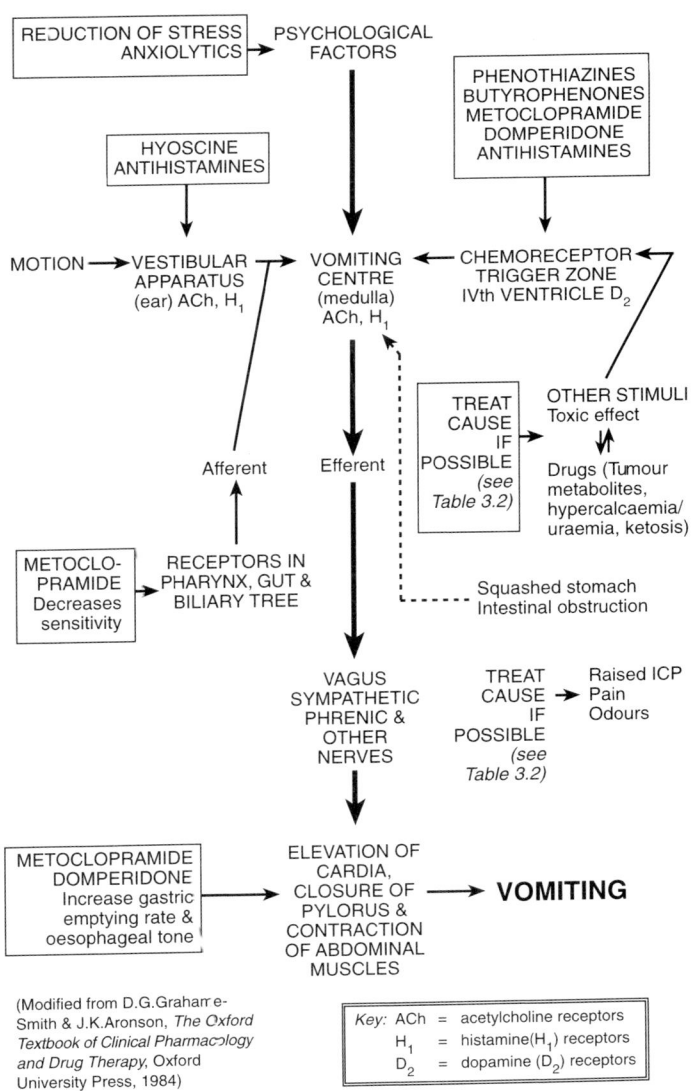

(Modified from D.G.Graham e-Smith & J.K.Aronson, *The Oxford Textbook of Clinical Pharmacology and Drug Therapy*, Oxford University Press, 1984)

| Key: | ACh | = | acetylcholine receptors |
|---|---|---|---|
| | $H_1$ | = | histamine($H_1$) receptors |
| | $D_2$ | = | dopamine ($D_2$) receptors |

**Figure 3.1** *Causes of nausea and vomiting*

**Table 3.1** *Causes of nausea and vomiting and their management*

| Cause | Antiemetic management |
|---|---|
| Psychological factors | Anxiolytic drugs: benzodiazepines, ?cannabinoids[†] |
| Vestibular disturbance | Belladonna alkaloids: hyoscine Antihistamines: cinnarizine[†] |
| Toxic effect on the chemoreceptor trigger zone | Dopamine antagonists: metoclopramide, domperidone |
| Abdominal causes | Metoclopramide, domperidone |
| Raised intracranial pressure | Dexamethasone[(a)] with an initial dose of 4 mg qid reducing to 4 mg bid. |

[(a)] Dexamethasone has many antiemetic effects possibly through cortical, emotional effect, appetite stimulation and reduction of pressure from tumour mass.

chemoreceptor zone is likely to respond to dopamine antagonists such as metoclopramide or domperidone.

*Management of nausea and vomiting*

Often simple measures such as removal of strong odours or the patient breathing through the open mouth may help. Sucking ice or sipping iced water or soda water is often helpful. Pharmacological management depends on the diagnosis of cause (Table 3.1) and treatment is shown in Table 3.2. Where possible, drugs should be given by mouth but if vomiting is present this route may not be tolerated. Domperidone may be given by suppository[†], hyoscine by skin patch, and dexamethasone, cyclizine hyoscine, and haloperidol may all be given sub-cutaneously via syringe driver. Where vomiting is severe it may be controlled with methotrimeprazine[†] 25–200 mg daily, if necessary subcutaneously by syringe driver; although this is effective it is also very sedative. Synthetic derivatives of cannabis such as Nabilone[†] offer promise with regard to control of vomiting associated with chemotherapy. Nabilone should be given orally in a dose of 1–2 mg bd (maximum 6 mg daily) starting the night before beginning cytotoxic treatment, and the second dose should be 1–3 hours before the first dose of the cytotoxic drug.

**Table 3.2** *Specific antiemetics, their indications and side-effects*

| Cause of nausea and vomiting | Antiemetic of choice and dose | Route | Side-effects |
|---|---|---|---|
| **Drug induced** | Haloperidol 1.5–3 mg nocte or. | Oral/s.c. | Side-effects unusual at lower dosage |
| | Fluphenazine 1–2 mg bid or. | Oral | |
| **Radiotherapy or chemotherapy** | Prochlorperazine 5 mg tid | Oral | |
| | Prochlorperazine 12.5 mg | i.m. | |
| | Prochlorperazine 25 mg | p.r. | |
| **Cytotoxic therapy** | Nabilone[+] 1–2 mg bd (max. 6 mg daily) throughout treatment cycle, ?ondansetron 4–8 mg od | Oral (start night before beginning cytotoxic therapy and second dose 1–3 hours before first dose of cytotoxic) | |
| **Metabolic: uraemia, hypercalcaemia** | Haloperidol 5–20 mg daily (Reduce plasma $Ca^{++}$ see pp. 40–41.) | Oral/s.c. | May cause dry mouth or drowsiness |
| **Raised intracranial pressure** | Dexamethasone 4 mg qid reducing to 4 mg bid | Oral/s.c. | Euphoriant |
| | Cyclizine 50–100 mg tid or qqh | Oral/i.m./i.v. | Causes drowsiness |
| | Hyoscine 300–600 μg tid | Oral/s.c. transdermal | Anticholinergic side-effects |
| **Intestinal obstruction** | Cyclizine 50–100 mg tid or qqh | Oral/i.m/i.v. | Causes drowsiness |
| | Hyoscine 400 μg tid | Oral/c.c. transdermal | Anticholinergic side-effects |
| | Methotrimeprazine[+][*] 12.5–25 mg | Oral/i.m/i.v. | Very sedative |
| | Methotrimeprazine 25–200 mg | s.c. | |
| **Oesoph. reflux Delayed gastric emptying** | Metoclopramide 10–20 mg tid/qqh | Oral/i.m/i.v. | May give rise to Parkinsonism |
| | Domperidone 10–20 mg tid/qqh | Oral | |
| | Domperidone 60 mg | p.r. | |

**Table 3.3** *Antiemetic compatibility in syringe*

| For subcutaneous infusion | Diamorphine† 10–50 mg/mL in 0.9% saline | |
|---|---|---|
| Compatible | Metoclopramide | 5 mg/mL |
| | Methotrimeprazine† | 10 mg/mL |
| | Hyoscine hydrobromide | 0.12 mg/mL |
| | Dexamethasone sodium phosphate | 1.6 mg/mL |
| Potentially incompatible | Haloperidol | 2 mg/mL |
| | Cyclizine lactate | 15 mg/mL |
| Incompatible | Chlorpromazine | 0.5 mg/mL |
| | Prochlorphenazine | 0.08 mg/mL |

In very severe vomiting, such as that induced by chemotherapeutic régimes including cisplatin, the new 5-$HT_3$ antagonist drug ondansetron (Zofran, Glaxo) is very effective; however, at £9 per 8 mg tablet it must be used with care. When using a syringe driver for pain control it is often convenient to give antiemetic drugs by the same route. Table 3.3 lists compatibility of antiemetic drugs with diamorphine in a syringe driver.

# Other upper gastrointestinal tract symptoms

*Halitosis and sore mouth*
Oral symptoms are common but are less often observed and treated. Drying of the mouth may be caused by mouth breathing, infection with candida or aphthous ulcers or drugs (especially cytotoxics and anti-cholinergics). Candida is probably present in most patients but is often overlooked. Bad breath may be due to poor hygiene, to pharyngeal cancer or infection and may also be caused by bronchial or upper gastrointestinal tract malignancy. Management depends on hygiene and care of dentures. Drying due to mouth breathing may be helped by encouraging fluids, sucking acid sweets or pineapple, or by the use of artificial saliva such as glandosane† (see Table 3.4), or an aerosol spray, which may be used to moisten the oropharynx. The use of

Table 3.4 *Drugs used for oral symptoms*

| Drug | Route | Dosage |
|------|-------|--------|
| Amphotericin | Oral | 100–200 mg four times daily |
| Artificial saliva (glandosane⁺) | Oral | Spray into mouth as required |
| Hydrocortisone | Oral | 2.5 mg lozenges four times daily |
| Ketoconazole | Oral | 200–400 mg daily |
| Metoclopramide | Oral | 10 mg thrice daily |
| Metronidazole | Oral | 0.2–1 g thrice daily |
| Nystatin | Oral | up to 500 000 units four times daily |

lemon and glycerine mouth swabs every 2 hours may be very helpful. If the symptom is very disturbing the patient's drugs should be checked for any with anticholinergic side-effects. Candida should be treated with oral nystatin suspension, amphotericin or ketoconazole. Aphthous ulcers may be helped by local application of hydrocortisone pellets. Halitosis caused by delay in gastric emptying due to cancer of the stomach may be helped by metoclopramide. The odour of oro-pharyngeal or bronchogenic cancer may be reduced with oral metronidazole.

## Anorexia

Anorexia is very common in advanced cancer and often does not worry patients as much as it does their relatives. Alcohol, in the patient's favourite form and served in appropriate glasses as a social event in the day rather than as yet another medicine provides calories, analgesia and may stimulate appetite. Drugs are rarely indicated for anorexia by itself though when there are other indications steroids, especially dexamethasone, markedly increase well-being and appetite.

## Loss of taste

Loss of taste in advanced cancer may be associated with zinc deficiency in those on inadequate diet or in protein-losing conditions. Deficiency of zinc produces an inability to taste zinc sulfate in 0.1% aqueous solution when patients are unable to distinguish the test from water. Zinc may be given as zinc sulfate (Zincaps or Solvazinc) 200 mg tid.

## Hiccup

Prolonged hiccupping, which may last for days, is exhausting, and painful. It may be caused mechanically, neurologically or chemically. Mechanical causes include direct diaphragmatic stimulus from irritation by tumour, infection or elevation of the diaphragm by ascites or hepatomegaly. Neurological causes include phrenic nerve irritation in the mediastinum from involvement in a hilar lung cancer. Hiccups may also be caused by tumours involving the central nervous system. Chemical causes are due to uraemia or to toxins from infection and occasionally from reduced levels of carbon dioxide due to overbreathing.

Treatment depends on diagnosis and removal of cause but in advanced cancer the causes are often refractory because of the presence of tumour or its metabolic effects. Stopping hiccups is not easy; popular remedies such as cold keys down the neck probably work, if at all, by reflex pharyngeal stimulation. Rebreathing from a paper bag is a simple means of correcting reduced $CO_2$ tension. Where there is gastric distension antiflatulent preparations such as asilone may be tried, metoclopramide may encourage gastric emptying and chlorpromazine (25 mg intravenously with a further 25 mg intramuscularly) often helps but may cause drowsiness and lightheadedness. In intractable hiccup baclofen 10 mg twice daily or nifedipine 20 mg thrice daily have been found helpful in some cases and are worth trying. In severe persistent hiccups surgical ablation of the phrenic nerve may have to be considered.

## Dysphagia

Dysphagia is commonly associated with cancer of the oesophagus or mouth but may be caused by pressure on the oesophagus from a mediastinal tumour and may also occur as a result of neurological disorders such as motor neurone disease or where the glosso-pharyngeal nerve is involved in the tumour. Candida may give rise to dysphagia especially in AIDS patients. It should be treated energetically with ketoconazole, although this may reduce the white count already depressed in immunodeficient patients. Extrinsic pressure from a mediastinal tumour may be relieved by dexamethasone or radiotherapy.

### The squashed stomach syndrome

This occurs when the stomach is prevented from distending by the enlargement of the liver or intra-abdominal masses and may also occur where surgery or tumour has reduced the size of the stomach. It gives rise to postprandial fullness, flatulence, hiccup and nausea. It may be treated with carminatives (e.g. cardamom, Asilone) and metoclopramide, 10 mg thrice daily, to hasten gastric emptying. Steroids may help by reducing tumour mass so relieving the pressure on the stomach.

### General comments

In all the symptom complexes discussed above, drugs are important but must always be used in conjunction with explanation, reassurance and optimism in an atmosphere of unhurried calm. In all cases this may be as therapeutic as the drug and without it the effect of the drug may be minimal.

## CHAPTER 4

# Other gastrointestinal symptoms

## Constipation

Individuals mean different things by the word constipation. To some it means failure of daily defaecation, to others merely a disturbance of far less regular habit. Constipation may mean the passing of hard scybalae or an inability to evacuate bulky soft faeces and, since these need different treatment, it is important to discover just what is meant by the terms embarrassed patients use to describe an altered state of bowel function. Constipation (see Table 4.1) is the commonest preventable problem of palliative care and often the most inadequately treated symptom of advanced cancer. Some 75–80% of patients treated in hospital or at home are grossly constipated, leading to many symptoms such as malaise, abdominal pain or vomiting. Constipation is inevitable where patients are receiving opioids unless care is taken to prevent it. Dyschezia may result from dietary deficiency, reduced fluid intake (this is especially important with bulk-forming aperients such as bran), inactivity, gastrointestinal disease or, most commonly, iatrogenically. *All* patients receiving palliative care should have attention paid to their bowel function and *all* prescriptions for opioids should be accompanied by aperients.

**Table 4.1** *Causes of constipation in patients with cancer*

- Reduced food intake particularly bulk-producing roughage foods
- Reduced fluid intake or, possibly, loss of fluid through excessive vomiting or sweating
- Immobility, which not only exacerbates constipation but prevents a patient from getting to the lavatory to answer the call to stool
- As a result of treatment, especially with opioids
- As a direct result of pelvic tumours

*Treatment*

Laxative drugs fall into four groups:

- Bulk-forming agents:    methylcellulose, bran, ispaghula, sterculia
- Osmotic laxatives:    magnesium sulfate (Epsom salts) lactulose*
- Faecal softeners:    arachis oil, liquid paraffin
- Stimulant laxatives:
  – anthracenes;    senna, fig, cascara, danthron†, docusate
  – polyphenols;    bisacodyl, sodium picosulfate.

A former proprietary favourite in Britain was Dorbanex liquid, which patients tolerated well but which was withdrawn because of rare side-effects. It is still available in Britain on a named patient basis for use in advanced cancer.

The first line of management is to perform a rectal examination on all patients with constipation. If the rectum is full of hard scybalae the patient should be given an arachis oil retention enema at night, followed the next morning by a phosphate enema. The patient may find this distressing but may be reassured by using soft incontinence pads to prevent embarrassment. If the

---

*Although lactulose has been included in this group it also acts as a bulk-forming agent. Lactulose, in addition to its osmotic effect, encourages colonic bacteria by acting as a substrate for these organisms, so increasing faecal mass.

**Table 4.2** *Treatment of constipation*

| | | |
|---|---|---|
| **Bulk formers** | | |
| • Ispaghula | Oral | 1–4 sachets/day |
| • Methylcellulose | Oral | 3–6 tabs/day |
| • Sterculia | Oral | 1–4 sachets/day |
| **Faecal softeners** | | |
| Arachis oil | Enema | |
| • Liquid paraffin | Oral | 10–30 mL/day |
| **Osmotic laxatives** | | |
| • Lactulose | Oral | 15 mL twice daily |
| • Magnesuium sulfate | Oral | 5–10 g/day |
| **Bowel stimulants** | | |
| • Bisacodyl | Oral | 10–20 mg/day |
| • Danthron⁺ | Oral | 1–3 caps/day |
| • Docusate | Oral | 100–500 mg/day |
| • Picosulfate sodium⁺ | Oral | 5–15 mL/day |
| • Senna | Oral | 2–4 tabs/day |
| **Enemas** | | |
| • Arachis oil retention enema | | 130 mL single disposable pack |
| • Phosphate enema | | Sodium acid phosphate 12.8 g and sodium phosphate 10.24 g in 128 mL water |
| • Micro enema | | Sodium citrate, sodium lauryl sulfate in single disposable packs |

rectum is empty and collapsed then there is no impaction. Usually this form of constipation responds to oral bulk formers given with plenty of fluid and peristaltic stimulants. An empty ballooned rectum indicates impacted faeces at the recto-sigmoid junction when lactulose accompanied by either senna or bisacodyl tablets may stimulate evacuation. If the mass collects in the lower rectum this will need treatment with either a phosphate or micro enema, with daily rectal assessment of the state of impaction until it is cleared. Once adequate bowel function is restored all patients on opioids will require a maintenance-dose oral aperient. Lactulose, starting with a dose of 15 mL twice daily is the drug of choice; the dose may be titrated up or down as required and a stimulant such as senna or bisacodyl may be required as well (see Table 4.2).

Table 4.3 *Treatment of diarrhoea*

| Drug | Route | Dosage |
|------|-------|--------|
| Kaolin | Oral | |
| Ispaghula | Oral | 1–4 sachets/day |
| Methylcellulose | Oral | 3–6 tabs/day |
| Sterculia | Oral | 1–4 sachets/day |
| Codeine phosphate | Oral | 10–300 mg/day |
| Diphenoxylate | Oral | 10 mg then 5 mg 4 hourly |
| Loperamide | Oral | 6–16 mg/day |
| Pancreatin | Oral | 1-2 caps thrice daily with food |

## Diarrhoea

Diarrhoea is an uncommon symptom that occurs in only about 4% of patients with advanced cancer (unless they have concomitant bowel disease such as ulcerative colitis). However, it is extremely common in the palliative care of people with AIDS. Loose motions result most commonly from spurious diarrhoea caused by faecal impaction. Steatorrhoea gives rise to fatty offensive floating stools and is associated with pancreatic insufficiency; it may respond to reduction of fat in the diet or to treatment with pancreatin which is inactivated by gastric acid and should be given with food. Diarrhoea may arise as part of a gastrointestinal upset usually of viral origin but may also be associated with a wide range of infections. The symptom is distressing to the patient since it is exhausting and carries with it associated anxiety about accidents and smells. This may be overcome if the mobile patient is nursed with easy access to the lavatory. Any call for commode or bedpan from immobile patients demands immediate response. The use of incontinence pads may give extra assurance but require frequent changing to prevent skin excoriation. Diarrhoea may be controlled with simple kaolin mixtures (see Table 4.3) although these are rarely adequate; sometimes sterculia, ispaghula or methylcellulose, more often used for constipation, will be helpful since they tend to bind loose stools and they may be particularly helpful in control of a colostomy or ileostomy. Antidiarrhoeal drugs that reduce motility such as codeine phosphate, diphenoxylate (Lomotil) and loperamide (Imodium) are particularly useful in the torrential diarrhoea due to crytosporidosis or isospora gut opportunistic infections seen in AIDS. Diphenoxylate may cause anticholinergic effects, especially dry mouth, and loperamide may cause rashes.

## Faecal incontinence

The most frequent cause of faecal incontinence, which is extremely distressing to both patient and relatives, is simply due to the accident of not being able to be in the right place at the right time. It may also be due to constipation, diarrhoea, to the presence of a pelvic cancer, to neurological disturbance of defaecation or to confusional states. In each case the underlying cause should be treated as far as possible. Faecal impaction with spurious diarrhoea is common, is frequently missed, and needs urgent treatment (*vide supra*). Where no remediable cause can be found the help of a continence adviser should be sought. She or he will advise on incontinence aids and the best way of helping the patient.

## Rectal symptoms

Rectal symptoms are common, uncomfortable and destructive of morale. They may be caused by faecal leakage, infection or tumour. Faecal leakage or incontinence may be due to lack of sphincter control as in paraplegia but may simply be due to spurious diarrhoea caused by constipation. Local perianal skin infection is often due to candida and will settle with canesten cream perhaps with added hydrocortisone. Rectal cancer may respond to palliative radiotherapy. Tenesmus is a particularly unpleasant rectal pain that is often markedly improved by chlorpromazine.

**Table** 4.4 *Medical treatment of intestinal obstruction*

| Drug | Route | Dosage |
|------|-------|--------|
| Cyclizine | Oral | 50 mg twice or thrice daily |
| Dexamethasone | Oral/s.c. | 2–16 mg/day |
| Docusate | Oral | 100–500 mg/day |
| Haloperidol | Oral | 5–10 mg/day |
| Hyoscine | Oral/s.c. | 400 µg thrice daily |
| Methotrimeprazine[†] | s.c. | 25–200 mg/day |
| Propantheline | Oral | 15 mg thrice daily |

## Intestinal obstruction

Where possible, intestinal obstruction should be treated surgically. Where this seems unjustifiable interference in a critically ill person then the condition may be treated conservatively (Table 4.4). Where the obstruction is low in the gastrointestinal tract the evacuation of the bowel by enema may help enormously. If the patient can tolerate aperients by mouth co-danthrusate[†] may help. It may also be possible to reduce the obstruction by shrinking the mass by reducing peritumoural oedema with dexamethasone up to 16 mg for a few days and then reducing to 4 mg daily.

Vomiting should be controlled as much as possible, preferably with oral preparations, or if necessary by syringe driver. First choice drugs are cyclizine or haloperidol, hyoscine may be useful as an antiemetic but is very drying to the mouth. In severe intractable cases methotrimeprazine (Nozinan)[†] may be given via a syringe driver but this is very sedative. Pain should be controlled with opioids or, if there is a great deal of spasmodic colicky pain, then antispasmodics should be given. In this context hyoscine is particularly useful since it is both antiemetic and antispasmodic; alternatively propantheline may be used.

Gastrointestinal symptoms are unpleasant enough by themselves but are also embarrassing and demoralising.

Good symptom control increases the patient's well-being and quality of life enormously. Despite this, insufficient attention is given to a patient's bowel function. Medicine, so clever at technology, is often let down by the mundane.

## CHAPTER 5

# Respiratory and central nervous system symptoms

## Respiratory symptoms

### Cough

Cough occurs in about one-third of patients with advanced cancer and in 80% of those with lung cancer. It may be caused by primary or secondary involvement of the lung with tumour, to secondary infection, to concurrent disease such as chronic obstructive lung disease, asthma or bronchiectasis or to smoking. Cough may be dry and irritant or productive. Dry cough is much more irritant and difficult to relieve. Search must be made for a removable cause. Bronchospasm requires bronchodilators by mouth or inhalation and infection may require antibiotics. (Where antibiotics are prescribed chloramphenicol is worth considering; it is an excellent antibiotic, which is rarely used in non-malignant patients because of exaggerated fears of bone marrow suppression and it can be very useful in palliative care.) The underlying cancer may need treatment with steroids, chemotherapy or radiotherapy, and physiotherapy and postural drainage should be considered. Dry cough may respond to humidification of the atmosphere with nebulised water to which salbutamol may be added if there is associated bronchospasm. Mucolytic drugs, such as acetylcysteine or carbocysteine[†], of little value in

Table 5.1 *Treatment of cough*

| Drug | Route | Dosage |
| --- | --- | --- |
| Acetylcysteine | Oral | 200 mg thrice daily |
| Carbocysteine⁺ | Oral | 0.75–1.5 g/day |
| Codeine linctus | Oral | 5–10 mL thrice daily |
| Diamorphine linctus⁺ | Oral | 2.5–10 mL 4 hourly |
| Methadone linctus⁺ | Oral | 2.5–5 mL 4 hourly |
| Salbutamol | Oral | 2–4 mg four times daily |
| | Inhaled | 2 puffs four times daily |
| | Nebulised | 2.5 mg four times daily |

treating non-malignant cough, may help where viscid sputum makes expectoration difficult. Cough medicines may help although most are little more effective than steam or cough sweets, which keep the upper respiratory tract moist. Where dry cough is exhausting, the use of linctuses of codeine, morphine⁺ or diamorphine⁺ may be indicated (see Table 5.1).

*Dyspnoea*
Like all other symptoms dyspnoea requires diagnosis. Although in most cases dyspnoea will be directly related to the cancer, other potentially remediable causes such as infection, heart failure or anaemia should be excluded. The management of this large and varied group of conditions is outside the scope of this book.

Dyspnoea is frightening and produces a vicious circle since fear worsens breathlessness. Dyspnoea occurs in about half of all cancer patients and in two-thirds of those with lung cancer. Patients are afraid that they will choke to death or stop breathing while asleep and should be reassured that neither will happen. Dyspnoea may be due to hyperventilation (when it will improve with re-breathing from a paper bag) or to heart failure, asthma, chest infection or pleural effusion. For those with no remediable cause the most important therapy is listening, explaining and reassuring.

Simple measures such as sitting the patient up, opening windows, the use of fans and breathing exercises

**Table** 5.2 *Treatment of dyspnoea amd haemoptysis caused by cancer*

| Drug | Route | Dosage |
|------|-------|--------|
| Dyspnoea | – | – |
| Diazepam | Oral | 2–5 mg thrice daily |
| Morphine | Oral/s.c | 2.5–5 mg 4 hourly |
| Haemoptysis | – | – |
| Diamorphine | Oral/s.c. | Related to previous dose |
| Diazepam | i.v. | 10–20 mg |

may be helpful as may distraction such as reading or television. In the absence of pain morphine orally or, if necessary subcutaneously, in small dosage (2.5–5 mg) may dramatically improve dyspnoea by reducing respiratory drive. Anxiolytic drugs such as diazepam may help enormously. Oxygen is less use than an open window. If the patient panics oral diazepam may be helpful but the most effective therapy is reassurance while the patient is held with a firm arm.

*Haemoptysis*
This is a frequent symptom of lung cancer and often very alarming to the patient. When caused by infection it may be eased with appropriate antibiotics. More often it is caused by the cancer and refractory to treatment. Patients require reassurance that they will not choke or bleed to death and may need sedation with diazepam or opioids. Severe bleeding as a terminal event is dealt with in Chapter 6.

Treatment of dyspnoea and haemoptysis is shown in Table 5.2.

# Central nervous system symptoms
*Insomnia*
Sleeplessness occurs in 30% of patients with advanced cancer. It may be due to failure of treatment for physical distress, fear, anxiety or depression and should be

Table 5.3 *Treatment of insomnia*

| Drug | Route | Dosage |
|------|-------|--------|
| Alcohol | Oral | Too much? too little? |
| Nitrazepam | Oral | 5–10 mg at night |
| Temazepam | Oral | 10–30 mg at night |
| Triazolam | Oral | 250 μg at night |

discussed in depth with the patient. All the patient's physical symptoms (especially nocturia) should be reviewed and treatment modified where necessary. Fear of dying during sleep may be so marked in some patients that they will fight to stay awake; here all that is needed may be reassurance and 'permission' to sleep. Insomnia is often subjective and mistaken for normal wakefulness and boredom. Under these circumstances reading or late night television may be all that is required. Only when alternatives have been tried should medication be prescribed since this may depress or sedate the patient. Alcohol may cause insomnia, either because of withdrawal or because it causes early waking. Benzodiazepines may be very helpful, particularly short acting drugs, such as temazepam. Drugs with a longer half-life, such as nitrazepam have the disadvantage of producing prolonged sedation and poor daytime concentration (see Table 5.3).

*Convulsions*

These may be due to pre-existing epilepsy or to primary or secondary brain cancer or to uraemia. Where patients are known to have widespread metastatic disease cerebral involvement may be assumed without further investigation, but in undiagnosed individuals fits indicate admission to hospital for brain scan. Convulsions are distressing for relatives, who should be warned of the possibility and instructed in first aid for patients known to have cerebral tumours. Fits should be controlled with 10 mg of intravenous diazepam, best given as diazemuls

**Table 5.4** *Treatment of convulsions*

| Drug | Route | Dosage |
| --- | --- | --- |
| Carbamazepine | Oral | 0.1–1.2 g/day |
| Diazepam | i./v. | 10–20 mg |
|  | p./r. | 10–20 mg |
| Dexamethasone | Oral/s.c. | 2–16 mg/day |
| Phenytoin | Oral | 100–600 mg/day |
| Sodium valproate | Oral | 0.6–2.5 g/day |

to prevent thrombophlebitis, or if this is impossible rectal diazepam may be used. The latter is very safe and some relatives may be trained to use it when immediate medical help is unavailable. Anticonvulsants such as phenytoin or carbamazepine should be prescribed and consideration given to the use of dexamethasone to reduce peritumoural oedema of cerebral masses (see Table 5.4).

*Weakness, lack of mobility and paralysis*

The increasing debility of advanced cancer produces many physical, psychological and social symptoms; common among these is an increasing lack of mobility. Weakness is so common in advanced cancer that it is easy to forget that there may be other and remediable causes such as overmedication, depression, boredom, lowered serum potassium, raised serum calcium, thyroid or suprarenal insufficiency. These should be considered in patients who feel weak although they are rarely responsible for it.

Paraplegia due to spinal metastases from breast, bronchus or prostatic primaries occurs in about 5% of cancer patients and may be preventable. The first symptom is usually pain, which may precede cord compression by anything from hours to years. Pain is usually felt at the site of the affected vertebra and may be worse on coughing or straining. There may be referred pain, paraesthesiae or weakness and there may be disturbance of sphincter function. The condition requires accurate diagnosis and immediate referral for

**Table 5.5** *Treatment of vertigo*

| Drug | Route | Dosage |
|------|-------|--------|
| Cinnazarine* | Oral | 30 mg thrice daily |
| Cyclizine | Oral | 50 mg bd or tid |
| Hyoscine | Oral/s.c. | 400 µg tid |
| Metoclopramide | Oral | 10 mg tid |

radiotherapy. Once paraplegia has developed due to metastatic cancer it is usually irreversible, though neurosurgical decompression should be considered.

*Vertigo and travel sickness*

Vertigo may occur in patients travelling to hospice day centres or to hospitals for treatment. Motion sickness can be controlled with hyoscine but this may produce unacceptable drying of the mouth. Antihistamines, such as cinnazarine† or cyclizine are useful, but metoclopramide and the phenothiazines, so useful in other forms of nausea, are ineffective in motion sickness. True vertigo may occur in coexistent Ménière's disease, in cerebral or eighth nerve tumours and following aural surgery. This may be difficult to manage but hyoscine, phenothiazines and antihistamines, in particular cinnazarine†, may be helpful (see Table 5.5).

*Restlessness*

This is worrying to relatives, particularly if combined with mild confusion, when patients may pick at their bedclothes (carphology — Greek, *karphos:* straw, *logeia:* gathering, also floccillation). Often the cause may be found in acute discomfort such as pain, a full bladder or rectum, and such cause should be searched for and treated appropriately. Only after the exclusion of physical causes should drugs be used. Every available help should be provided including night care (in Britain from Marie Curie nurses or the night watch service available from some social service departments).

**Table 5.6** *Causes of confusion*

1. **Unfamiliar stimuli:**
   - Too hot or cold
   - Discomfort in bed
   - Full bladder or rectum
   - Pain, pruritus, nausea, dehydration

2. **Change in environment:**
   - Leaving home
   - Changing bed position
   - Loss of known ward neighbours

3. **Metabolic disturbance:**
   - Uraemia
   - Hypercalcaemia
   - Hypoxia
   - Hyponatraemia
   - Hypoglycaemia
   - Hepatic failure
   - Toxaemia of sepsis
   - Deficiency states (vitamin, hormone)

4. **Tumour-induced insufficiency:**
   - Systemic effect
   - Cerebral involvement
   - Intracranial haemorrhage

5. **Psychiatric disorders:**
   - Depression
   - Anxiety
   - Schizo-affective disorders
   - Schizophrenia

6. **Drug induced:**
   - Narcotics
   - Phenothiazines
   - Antiparkinsonian drugs
   - Barbiturates
   - Digoxin
   - $H_2$ blockers
   - Benzodiazepines

7. **Drug withdrawal:**
   - Alcohol
   - Opioids
   - Barbiturates
   - Benzodiazepines

8. **Other cerebral diseases:**
   - Alzheimer's disease
   - Cerebrovascular
   - Dementia, AIDS etc.

9. **Intercurrent infections:**
   - Especially those of chest and bladder

## Confusion

This common problem of the very ill requires great care in diagnosis. Confusion may manifest itself in any combination of symptoms such as lack of concentration, loss of short-term memory, disorientation in time or space, misperceptions, paranoid delusions, hallucinations, rambling speech, restlessness, and aggressive or noisy behaviour.

Physical impairment such as deafness, anxiety or pain may mimic confusion and it is important to exclude these before assuming that a patient is confused. Causes of confusion are listed in Table 5.6.

Management of confusion depends on the removal of cause wherever possible, with as much explanation to the patient and relatives as possible, stressing that the patient

**Table 5.7** *Treatment of confusion*

| Drug | Route | Dosage |
|------|-------|--------|
| Chlormethiazole | Oral | 4–6 x 250 mg/day |
| Dexamethasone | Oral/s.c. | 2–16 mg/day |
| Haloperidol | Oral/s.c. | 1–30 mg/day |
| Methotrimeprazine | s.c.[†] | 25–200 mg/day |
| Thioridazine | Oral | 100–600 mg/day |

is not becoming insane. Restraint should be avoided and drugs, which are quite as likely to be the cause rather than the cure, should continually be reviewed with minimal medication where possible. In cerebral tumours dexamethasone may be indicated and haloperidol, thioridazine or chlormethiazole may help but again should be reviewed early and withdrawn if not beneficial. Thioridazine syrup is well tolerated and particularly useful because it is easy to titrate against the patient's confusion in order to control without oversedation. Methotrimeprazine[†] is very sedative but may be required in severe cases. Dosages of these drugs are shown in Table 5.7.

## CHAPTER 6

# Other physical symptoms

## Skin problems

### Excessive sweating

This common symptom of advanced cancer may be due to overheating since many wards are too hot and bedclothes may be heavy or of inappropriate material. Sweating may be caused by respiratory or urinary infection but may also be caused by the tumour itself. An $H_2$ blocker (e.g. cimetadine 200 mg) at night may help. Excessive sweating may sometimes be relieved by paracetamol, non-steroidal anti-inflammatory agents (e.g. indomethacin) or by small doses of a $\beta$-blocker (e.g. propranolol) (see Table 6.1).

### Pruritus

This may result from pre-existing skin disease but there may be a dry flaking of skin in advanced cancer or skin maceration from incontinence. The source of itching may be the nightclothes, which should be made of cotton. Drug reactions should always be considered and occasionally there may be psychogenic causes. Pruritus may be caused by cancer, as in Hodgkin's disease or melanomatosis, or because of secondary metabolic effects such as jaundice or uraemia. Itching may respond to simple measures such as keeping the patient cool. Management consists of scrupulous attention to skin hygiene; washing is particularly important in uraemia,

Table 6.1 *Treatment of excessive sweating*

| Drug | Route | Dosage |
|------|-------|--------|
| Cimetidine | Oral | 200 mg thrice daily |
| Indomethacin[a] | Oral | 25 mg thrice daily |
| Paracetamol | Oral | 0.5–1 g 4 hourly |
| Propranolol[a] | Oral | 10–40 mg thrice daily |

[a] May be given as a single daily dose in slow release preparations (i.e. Indocid R, Inderal LA) where these are available.

when patients may excrete irritant urea and bile salts in sweat, the so-called urea frost. Drugs are more often the cause than the cure of pruritus but may be needed (see Table 6.2). The pruritus of obstructive jaundice may be responsive to haloperidol, to steroids, such as dexamethasone or stanozolol, or to testosterone. Cholestyramine, often quoted in textbooks, is unpleasant to take and not recommended. A popular hospice remedy is cucumber liquidised in a household blender and applied to the skin.

## Fungating/bleeding skin tumours

These cause distress because of odour, pain or disfigurement. The lesions may be cleansed and dressed with hydrogen peroxide or 4% povidone-iodine compounds such as Betadine 1 part to 4 parts of liquid paraffin. Charcoal dressings sometimes relieve odour and metronidazole may be very useful by mouth or applied as a gel to the fungating lesion. Capillary bleeding from

Table 6.2 *Treatment of pruritus*

| Drug | Route | Dosage |
|------|-------|--------|
| Dexamethasone | Oral/s.c. | 2–16 mg/day |
| Cholestyramine | Oral | 4–8 g/day |
| Haloperidol | Oral | 0.5 mg thrice daily or 2 mg at night |
| Methyltestosterone | Oral | 10 mg thrice daily |
| Stanozolol | Oral | 5 mg/day |

fungating tumours is distressing and may be lessened by the use of dressings soaked in 1:1000 adrenalin.

*Decubitus ulcers*

Care of patients' skin is important since pressure sores can lead to further pain and discomfort. The old adage 'you may put anything on a pressure area but the patient' is very true. Regular changes of position, at least every 2 hours. are needed whether the patient is in bed all the time or sitting in a chair. Aids such as Spenco mattresses and cushions, sheepskins, or waterbeds, are merely adjuncts to such positional change. Although these aids have an important role when correctly used they are only part of care. Good handling and lifting techniques are also important because when poorly carried out may lead to shearing of the patient's skin and subsequent sores. Sources of potential trauma, such as watches, rings and long fingernails should be dealt with.

# Urinary symptoms

Urinary symptoms include increased frequency or urgency of micturition due to detrusor instability. Bladder spasm may be caused by concentration (which predisposes to infection) of urine in patients whose fear of dysuria makes them frightened to drink adequately. Infection in the catheterised patient should be treated with normal saline bladder washouts or urinary antiseptics such as chlorhexidine but non-catheterised patients require appropriate antibiotics. Bladder spasm may respond to anticholinergic drugs such as propantheline, amitryptiline or terodiline[+] but if their side-effects are troublesome then flavoxate (Urispas) may help. Retention may be due to benign or malignant prostatic enlargement, drugs (especially anticholinergic drugs such as tricyclic antidepressants), neurological causes or be precipitated by a full rectum. Retention may by relieved by immersion of the patient in a hot bath but most patients need catheterisation. Urinary incontinence

Table 6.3 *Treatment of urinary symptoms*

| Drug | Route | Dosage |
|------|-------|--------|
| Amitriptyline | Oral | 25–75 mg twice daily |
| Chlorhexidine | Bladder washout (some advocate normal saline) | |
| Flavoxate | Oral | 200 mg thrice daily |
| Propantheline | Oral | 15–30 mg thrice daily |
| Terodiline' | Oral | 12.5–25 mg twice daily |

obviously affects the quality of a patient's life and priority of care for each patient must be to maintain and promote self-esteem. It is important to ascertain the reason for incontinence and if possible treat it. Each patient must be examined to exclude underlying pathology or inappropriate medication. Faecal impaction is a common cause in patients who are receiving opioids. If the patient is at home it may be that the toilet is difficult to reach. The loan of a commode and/or urinals may be arranged through the community nurse. The provision of a raised toilet seat and hand rails may help patients with limited mobility. Patients and relatives may find it difficult to talk about incontinence so the caring team need a sympathetic but matter-of-fact approach. Appropriate incontinence aids should be supplied and the local authority laundry service and continence adviser may be involved. In the final stages of the patient's illness it may be kinder to catheterise the patient in order to prevent persistent wet beds. Where catheter care is needed for a male patient, a condom-type appliance such as a convene may be useful (see Table 6.3).

# Metabolic disturbance

*Hypercalcaemia*
Hypercalcaemia occurs in about 10–20% of cases of advanced cancer. Though it may occur in association with many primary tumours, those in the lung, breast and

Table 6.4 *Treatment of hypercalcaemia*

| Drug | Route | Dosage |
|------|-------|--------|
| Dexamethasone | Oral/s.c. | 2–16 mg/day |
| Frusemide | Oral | 40 mg/day |
| Mithramycin | Oral | 25 µg/kg |
| Sodium cellulose phosphate | Oral | 5 g thrice daily |
| Pamidronate | i.v. (well diluted in calcium-free i.v. infusion) | Dosage determined by plasma calcium levels |

kidney give rise to aberrant parathormone-like substances most frequently. Multiple myelomatosis also may cause hypercalcaemia. Mild elevation of serum calcium up to about 2.8 mmol/L rarely causes symptoms, but above this patients suffer worsening of all their previous symptoms particularly nausea, vomiting, confusion, pain and constipation. In severe instances there may be dehydration and increasing confusion leading to coma. Above 3.5 mmol/L it is unlikely that any treatment will be helpful.

Mild hypercalcaemia is treated by producing diuresis with frusemide and extra fluids (see Table 6.4). At the same time steroid therapy with dexamethasone 4 mg bd is recommended. If this is ineffective then sodium cellulose phosphate tablets (Calcisorb) will help to bind calcium in the gut but should not be given if the serum phosphate is unduly raised. Formerly mithramycin 25 µg/kg was given by slow intravenous infusion but this has been superseded by chelating agents such as pamidronate (Aredia) also given by slow intravenous infusion in a dose related to the blood calcium level. In the severe hypercalcaemia of advanced cancer the decision to start active aggressive therapy may be difficult and it will depend on the patient's general state and willingness to tolerate unpleasant treatment.

*Uraemia*

Uraemia is a common late event with many cancers especially those affecting the urinary tract. There is often little that can be done for it but the complications of thirst, drowsiness, skin irritation and pericarditis may be troublesome and require symptomatic relief.

## Terminal care

When palliative care has been conducted well the emphasis of care at the end may shift from the patient to the family. The strain of caring for a loved close relative at home is enormous. Such strain can be borne more easily where relatives feel themselves members of the nursing and medical team and a few words of encouragement and praise from a respected doctor or nurse can give carers new heart. For the doctor there can be few tasks so satisfying as well conducted care of a family through such a death.

It is important to appreciate the difference between palliative and terminal care. Palliative care begins with the decision that cure is no longer possible but it is wrong to call this terminal care with its overtones of hopelessness. The very essence of palliative care is hope for maximum quality of life, sometimes for many years. Terminal care is agonal, involving the last days or hours of the patient's life. The change from palliative care to terminal care is not easy to define since both are concerned with the quality of remaining life. There comes a point, however, when further active treatment designed to improve quality of life may actually diminish it. Here one comes into difficult transitional areas since some may argue that to withhold treatment that could prolong life is tantamount to euthanasia. Euthanasia (Greek: *eu* good, *thanatos* death) is a much misused word, which really means good death but has come to mean 'assisted death'. There is an artificial division of such action into active euthanasia (i.e. deliberate killing) and passive euthanasia (the withholding of a drug or procedure that might prolong life but in the opinion of the carer would unbearably reduce the quality of life). The former, in the writer's opinion, is unacceptable and absence of the latter inhumane.

### Symptoms in terminal care

There comes a time when, in the presence of terminal infection, haemorrhage, confusion, convulsions, respiratory failure or profound metabolic disturbance, treatment should be aimed at improving the quality of what life remains rather than merely prolonging it. A good rule is to ask oneself whether the proposed treatment would distress the patient more than the symptoms it aims to ameliorate. In such a decision the views of relatives and other members of the clinical team should be considered.

### Respiratory problems

Terminal pneumonia, often referred to as 'the old man's friend', rarely responds to antibiotics and their prescription serves only to prolong the agony for patient and relatives. The difficulty comes in deciding when such pneumonia is in fact terminal rather than an intercurrent episode in what may, thanks to good palliative care, be a long period of enjoyable life of high quality. A late symptom that is often very distressing to relatives and to other patients is the noisy terminal respiration that occurs near death. The tachypnoea that often occurs may be slowed with intravenous diamorphine and the noise, the so-called death rattle, may be eased and quietened with hyoscine.

### Haemorrhage

Very rarely there may be mediastinal haemorrhage sufficient to cause acute tracheal obstruction when death may be immediate; where there is acute distress diazepam should be administered intravenously. Exsanguinating haemorrhage is fortunately very rare but when it occurs is very frightening to the patient, relatives and other patients. It may occur due to rupture of a large vessel into a main bronchus, the stomach, rectum or vagina. When the bleeding is arterial death is very rapid but in the commoner venous bleeding it may be slow and terrifying. Intravenous sedation is required with diazepam and/or diamorphine. The quantity of blood lost can be very frightening to onlookers and the availability of red towels and blankets will help to minimise distress. Following such an event there will be a need of support for all the medical and nursing staff involved. Relatives witnessing such a death may require long-term counselling.

*Terminal confusion*

This can be extremely distressing to exhausted relatives since it appears that the patient is suffering. When additional sedation is necessary methotrimeprazine[†] by syringe driver will ensure a more peaceful end. Similarly, severe convulsions due to cerebral lesions or to uraemia will require sedation, usually via syringe driver, when combinations of opioids and methotrimeprazine may be more satisfactory than conventional anticonvulsants.

Severe hypercalcaemia is another condition in which it may be appropriate to treat the patient symptomatically since intravenous lines, frequent venesection and the administration of drugs such as pamidronate may be intolerable for the patient.

## CHAPTER 7

# Psychological problems

## Anxiety

Anxiety is present to some degree or other in almost all patients with advanced cancer. To the patient the disease is a new experience for which he has no yardstick of normality. The carer's knowledge of what may happen is vital to the anxious patient. Once having accepted the diagnosis of cancer a patient may attribute every new and trivial symptom to the cancer and assume that the condition is worsening. As a young patient dying of melanomatosis put it: 'The fear of cancer is worse than cancer'. Thus patients need listening time more than anything else, followed by detailed reassurance about their problems. Patients often want to know what may happen to them and turn to their carers as experts in death and dying to ask how they will end. Particular fears concern pain, choking in those who are dyspnoeic and severe haemorrhage in those who are bleeding. These questions can be difficult particularly where the fear may be justified.

Drug treatment of anxiety has earned itself a justifiably bad name since in the past it has often been found easier to prescribe than to listen and explain. However, anxiolytic drugs have a place in palliative care after appropriate listening and counselling. Choice of drug may depend on the patient's other medication, which may include phenothiazines or hypnotics.

Sometimes it may be more appropriate to adjust dosage of other medication rather than prescribe additional anxiolytics. The benzodiazepines are among the most useful drugs. Diazepam may be given orally, rectally or intravenously and is rapid in action but does tend to sedate. Lorazepam is available for oral or intravenous administration and lorazepam tablets are absorbed rapidly sublingually. Opioids are probably the best anxiolytics.

*Management of anxiety*

1. Sit so that your eyes are at the same level as the patient's. Listen attentively and be seen to understand the patient's fear.
2. Reassure about the patient's unrealistic fears.
3. Minimise fears that may have substance but without belittling them, for patients will not be helped if their anxiety is not being taken seriously.
4. Remove relievable physical symptoms wherever possible, especially hyperventilation.
5. Touch the patient. Touching is most important when reassuring frightened people. In severe panic attacks the firm holding of a patient in the carer's arms may be very helpful.
6. Seek recourse to anxiolytic drugs only after all the previous techniques have been followed.

# Depression

Depression is difficult to define and classify. There are four main concepts covered by the term.[1]

1. *Reaction to life situation.* Patients complain of depression and misery consequent upon unhappiness relating to their illness, disturbed relationships, or because of adverse social or financial situations. Such factors are common in cancer patients and may be contributory to, or exacerbate, reactive or endogenous depression.

2. *Reactive depression.*   This is the depression caused by major, usually single, identifiable, personal disasters such as loss of loved ones, pets or property. Patients facing imminent death frequently grieve over their anticipated loss.

3. *Endogenous depression.*   This form of depression wells up from within the individual, lacks identifiable causative adverse life events (though it may be associated with serious debilitating physical disease or major surgery) and is associated with self-criticism, anhedonia, a lack of future, and suicidal thought, which in cancer patients may be expressed in a request for euthanasia. Endogenous depression is characterised by retardation of physical function, especially bowel and sexual activity and alteration of sleep patterns with early morning waking.

4. *Schizo-affective disorders.* Severe disorders of emotion may be associated with disorders of cognition similar to, but falling short of, true schizophrenia. This is rare in palliative care except where the psychiatric condition antedates the cancer.

A single patient may show any mixture of these concepts. Depression is commonly associated with physical illness; as many as 25% of individuals with severe physical illness are also clinically depressed.

Depression is probably caused by disturbance in the metabolism of neurotransmitters including nor-adrenalin, dopamine, γ-amino-butyric acid (GABA), and serotonin or 5-hydroxy tryptamine (5-HT) within the limbic system. Depression is thought to result from cholinergic, and mania from adrenergic, predominance. Endogenous depression appears to be associated with altered metabolism of 5-HT in the central nervous system. There are multiple 5-HT receptors in the brain, where it is thought antidepressant drugs may block serotonin uptake. Depression may also be a side-effect of

Table 7.1 *Treatment of depression*

| Drug | Route | Dosage |
|------|-------|--------|
| Amitriptyline | Oral | 50–200 mg/day |
| Dexamphetamine† | Oral | 5–15 mg/day |
| Imipramine | Oral | 75–200 mg/day |
| Tranylcypromine | Oral | 10–20 mg/day |
| Maprotiline† | Oral | 25–150 mg/day |
| Mianserin | Oral | 30–200 mg/day |
| Phenelzine | Oral | 30–60 mg/day |

anticonvulsants, clonidine, phenothiazine, methyldopa, reserpine and other drugs, and benzodiazepines and other anxiolytic drugs may actually worsen depression.

*Management of depression*

In all cases management involves listening, counselling and perhaps referral to social services and other agencies. Drug therapy is required in a minority who show evidence of marked pathological depression usually of endogenous origin. Many forms of depression respond to treatment other than with drugs. Treatment may include any, or all of, simple psychotherapy, social manipulation, family counselling and drugs; drugs used to treat depression are listed in Table 7.1.

Drug therapy plays little or no part in the management of unhappiness consequent upon a poor life situation. Sometimes minor tranquillisers may be required in crisis but anxiolytic drugs are *not* antidepressants and their use in undiagnosed endogenous depression may make it worse. In reactive depression drug therapy plays only a minor role in most cases but antidepressants may be needed where the reaction is prolonged or fails to respond to listening and counselling.

Though the natural history of endogenous depression is one of slow improvement in palliative care it may reduce the quality of the patient's life. Tricyclic antidepressants are the drugs of first choice although the newer tetracyclics (e.g. maprotiline†, mianserin) may be indicated because of less side-effect or cardio-toxicity. In schizo-affective disorders the use of antidepressant drugs may need to be supplemented with major or minor tranquillisers.

Of the drugs available for treatment of depression tricyclic antidepressants are the most effective and are of two main types:

- Dibenzapines: including imipramine, desipramine, trimipramine, clomipramine, iprindole[†], opipramol[†], dibenzapin[†].
- Dibenzocycloheptenes: including amitriptyline, nortriptyline, protriptyline, butriptyline[†], doxepin, dothiepin.

Some drugs have an immediate sedative effect, which may be very useful since many depressed patients are severely sleep depleted as a result of prolonged early morning waking. Dosage of tricyclic antidepressants is critical since there appears to be a relatively narrow therapeutic window, above or below which optimum response does not occur. With most antidepressants relief of depression may not become apparent for 3 weeks, which may be inappropriate for very ill patients.

Anticholinergic side-effects such as dry mouth, constipation and blurred vision may be troublesome in palliative care. Side-effects may be less marked if the patient is started on a small dose, which is gradually increased every 3 to 4 days. A single dose given at night may also help patients to tolerate side-effects. Because of their marked anticholinergic effect caution should be observed when treating patients with incipient glaucoma or prostatism. Retarded and anergic patients may be helped by drugs with more stimulant action such as desipramine or clomipramine. Tricyclics may lower the convulsive threshold and must be used with caution in patients prone to fits.

Monoamine oxidase inhibitors (e.g. tranylcypromine, phenelzine) are less effective and more dangerous than tricyclics and there may be interactions with tyramine-containing foods and with tricyclic antidepressants, pethidine, phenothiazines, reserpine, sympathomimetics, antihypertensives and general anaesthetics.

Amphetamines[†] still have a place in the treatment of depression in palliative care since the risk of dependence in patients with a poor prognosis is small. Dexamphetamine has an advantage over tricyclics antidepressants since its antidepressant effect is almost immediate. Steroids have euphoriant properties and, though not advocated as treatment for depression, may relieve it when prescribed for other reasons.

## Care of carers

Palliative care is perhaps the most emotionally exacting form of therapy. Carers are continually exposed to highly stressful experiences and ethical dilemmas. The highly supportive nature of care puts a heavy burden on all medical, nursing and other caring staff, which may reach a peak with young or particularly disturbing deaths. This means that there has to be a network of concern among all who work in this field such that each is aware of stress in the others and is prepared to listen to and where necessary counsel colleagues across professional boundaries.

## CHAPTER 8

# AIDS—a special problem of palliative care

IN much of Africa, AIDS affects women as much as men. It is estimated that throughout the world some 8–10 million people have the human immunodeficiency virus (HIV), of which about 5 million are men and 3 million women. In North America and Europe AIDS is predominantly a disease of homosexual and bisexual males (see Table 8.1), but it is slowly spreading into the heterosexual population. In the year September 1989 to 1990 AIDS cases acquired through heterosexual intercourse rose from 123 to 240 (a 95% increase) while cases acquired through IVD abuse showed an increase of 89% and those acquired among male homosexual or bisexual men increased by 41%. During that year HIV-positive tests have risen by 57% in heterosexuals and by 41% in male homosexual/bisexuals. In Britain during the year to September 1993 male AIDS cases increased by 2% while female numbers went up by 43% and reports of AIDS acquired through sex between men and women increased by 12%.

An important bridge between homosexual and heterosexual groups is made up by intravenous drug users particularly where prostitution is used to finance the habit. In America the increasingly popular drug 'crack' is increasing the spread of the virus alarmingly. Recent

**Table 8.1** *AIDS in the United Kingdom — cases and deaths by means of exposure (Jan. 1982–Sep. 1993)[1]*

| Transmission category | Males | Deaths | Females | Deaths | Total | Deaths |
|---|---|---|---|---|---|---|
| **Sexual intercourse** | | | | | | |
| • Between men | 6043 | 3930 | – | – | 6043 | 3930 |
| • Between men and women: | | | | | | |
|   high risk partner | 26 | 13 | 68 | 37 | 94 | 50 |
|   other partner abroad | 415 | 219 | 258 | 102 | 673 | 321 |
|   other partner UK | 43 | 19 | 34 | 18 | 77 | 37 |
|   under investigation | 7 | 4 | 3 | 1 | 10 | 5 |
| • All heterosexual transmission | 491 | 255 | 363 | 158 | 854 | 413 |
| **Injecting drug use (IDU)** | 282 | 167 | 122 | 70 | 404 | 237 |
| **IDU or sex between men** | 132 | 85 | – | – | 132 | 85 |
| **Blood** | | | | | | |
| • Blood factor (e.g. for haemophilia) | 375 | 304 | 6 | 4 | 381 | 308 |
| **Tissue transfer** (e.g. transfusion) | | | | | | |
| • Abroad | 11 | 6 | 34 | 20 | 45 | 26 |
| • UK | 19 | 16 | 23 | 20 | 42 | 36 |
| **Mother to infant** | 46 | 22 | 53 | 26 | 99 | 48 |
| **Other/undetermined** | 97 | 59 | 18 | 11 | 115 | 70 |
| **Total** | 7496 | 4844 | 619 | 309 | 8115 | 5153 |

It is estimated that the real total of HIV infected persons in UK could be between 50 000 and 100 000.
*Source:* Communicable Disease Surveillance Centre 1993

trends suggest that a similar effect is occurring in Britain. Although smoked, and so not a means of direct transfer, 'crack' leads to sexual hyperactivity leading to the spread of sexually transmitted diseases (STD) including HIV. Long-term studies suggest that transfer of the virus from men to women is greater than from women to men. About 25% of women cohabiting with infected men become infected and about 10% of males having regular sex with infected women become seropositive.[2] The spread of the virus is greatly increased by the presence of other STDs, particularly herpes and syphilis, which produce genital ulcers so allowing viral entry to the recipients' blood.

Blood and its products used in the treatment of haemophilia, formerly a cause of infection, are now safe.

## The virus

The human immunodeficiency virus (HIV) belongs to a group of RNA viruses known as retroviruses, which possess the enzyme reverse transcriptase. This enzyme enables viral RNA to be inserted into the DNA of the nucleus of the host lymphocyte so converting the cell into a factory for the manufacture of more virus. Retroviruses are very highly specialised and, in consequence, extremely fragile and easily destroyed by heating to 56°C for 30 minutes or by simple chemical disinfectants such as bleach.

It must be stressed that the human immunodeficiency virus is extremely fragile and difficult to catch unless there is direct transfusion of lymphocytes containing the virus into the blood stream of a recipient. Lymphocytes obviously occur in blood; there are also many lymphocytes in semen. These two fluids are the most dangerous from the point of view of infection, which takes place during blood to blood or semen to blood contact. Semen to blood contact can occur sexually where there is a break in the mucous membrane of the organ in which ejaculation occurs whether it is vagina, rectum or mouth. The virus has been isolated from many body fluids but infection is only a risk from fluids containing blood cells. Thus any blood-stained body fluid is a hazard as are CSF, fluid from peritoneal, pleural, pericardial or synovial effusions, amniotic fluid or vaginal secretions, which should all be handled with the same precautions as blood. Saliva is generally safe except during dentistry, where it may be contaminated with blood. Unfixed tissue is also a hazard. Transmission may occur vertically across the placenta or rarely during breast feeding.

Extreme care must be taken when handling potentially infected blood during surgery, venesection or in the laboratory. Blood suspected of being infected with

HIV should be sent to the laboratory with full biohazard precautions. Accidental spillage of blood should be flooded with hypochlorite solutions containing 10 000 parts per million of available chlorine, and clothing contaminated with blood or semen should be autoclaved.

The possibility of health-care workers becoming infected by accidental needle-stick injuries is a common cause of concern. Up to 1988, 26 health-care workers throughout the world have been reported as becoming HIV-positive without identifiable non-occupational risk. When one considers the enormous number of medical and nursing personnel who have been involved in the care of potentially infected patients this number is minute. In the United States the surveillance project of the Center for Disease Control has estimated the risk of seroconversion after a single accidental needle-stick at less than 0.5% compared with a risk of 20% for transmission of the Hepatitis B virus.

When a person suspected of having HIV or hepatitis dies undertakers and others who may handle the body must be informed of potential risk of infection. This may appear to contravene the strict code of confidentiality imposed on all health-care workers, especially those working in contact with people with AIDS, but it must be remembered that the label 'danger of infection' is required in a number of other diseases such as haemorrhagic fevers and hepatitis. Death certification may pose problems of confidentiality. In Britain this may be overcome by recording that more information can be obtained by initialling the appropriate box on the certificate so that recorders can approach the certifying doctor for confidential information for statistical and epidemiological purposes.

## The clinical picture

Seroconversion usually occurs between 6 weeks and 6 months after infection with HIV (but may be delayed indefinitely) and may be associated with a febrile illness

**Table 8.2** *Incidence of diseases occurring in AIDS patients*

| Disease | Incidence (%) |
| --- | --- |
| *Pneumocystis carinii* pneumonia (PCP) | 63 |
| Kaposi's sarcoma (KP) | 24 |
| Candidiasis | 14 |
| Cytomegalovirus infection | 7 |
| Cryptococcosis | 7 |
| Chronic Herpes simplex | 4 |
| Cryptosporidiosis | 4 |
| Isosporiasis | 3 |
| Toxoplasmosis | 3 |
| Other opportunistic infection | 3 |

These figures are probably an underestimate since many patients have multiple infection.

similar to infectious mononucleosis but which may be so mild as to be unnoticed by the patient. In some individuals there may be no further development for many years or there may be progression to the AIDS related complex (ARC) or persistent generalised lymphadenopathy (PGL) associated with fever, night sweats, malaise and weight loss. Progression from either of these HIV related states may occur, with the development of the full syndrome. Data from San Francisco suggests that progression from seropositivity to full blown AIDS is variable and slow but that 50% of seropositive individuals will develop AIDS within 10 years. More recent data suggest that this figure may be as high as 60% by 7 years.[2] As with many data regarding AIDS there are widely disparate figures; the truth is that the full extent of the disease is not known for certain. The characteristic feature of AIDS is impaired immunity, which manifests itself in opportunistic infection or unusual forms of malignancy. Opportunistic infections (OI) include many viral, bacterial, fungal and protozoan diseases that are normally rare in immunocompetent individuals (see Table 8.2).

## Treatment

The process by which reverse transcriptase encodes the RNA of HIV into the DNA of the host lymphocyte requires thymidine; zidovudine (see Table 8.3) acts by mimicking thymidine so inhibiting the insertion of viral RNA in the host cell nucleus. There is some evidence that zidovudine (formerly azidothymidine, AZT) produces symptomatic improvement in people with AIDS but probably does little for long-term prognosis. This raises important ethical questions about the treatment of the syndrome, for zidovudine is expensive (a week's treatment used to cost about £120 or £6000 a year for drugs alone but a newly recommended reduced dose has lowered this to £60 a week or £3000 a year). With the ever increasing numbers of patients it is easy to see that the cost of treating AIDS patients could exhaust resources to such an extent that there would be little left for other diseases. This in no way belittles the AIDS patients' need for care but it must be realised that patients suffering from other diseases have equal right to treatment.

As there is no cure for AIDS all care is in effect palliative and differs little from the palliative care of cancer — good communication and symptom control are essential. Counselling is complicated by the critical attitude of society towards AIDS, because of the youth of people with AIDS and because the possibility of dementia and crossinfection cause special problems.

Counselling has two main aims. First it aims to reduce the spread of HIV through the alteration of sexual practices and the encouragement of monogamy, few sexual partners or safer sex. Secondly it aims to minimise the psychological effect and consequences of being infected with the virus. Counselling is also needed prior to and, where the result is positive, after HIV testing. This can be fraught with ethical difficulty. It is important to explain that testing for seroconversion is not a test for AIDS, that a negative test does not guarantee freedom from infection, and to discuss the implications of a

Table 8.3 *Drugs used in HIV-related disease*

| Indication | Drug name | Route | Dose range | Important side-effects |
|---|---|---|---|---|
| Helicoobacter | Erythromycin | Oral | 250–500 mg 6 hourly | GIT symptoms |
| Candida | Amphotericin | Oral i.v. | 100–200 mg 4 times daily 250 µg/kg/day | GIT symptoms, renal toxicity, cardiotoxicity, neurological symptoms |
| | Ketoconazole | Oral | 200–400 mg daily | Hepatotoxicity, reduction of white cells |
| | Nystatin | Oral | Up to 500 000 units four times daily | GIT symptoms |
| Cytomegalovirus | Ganciclovir | i.v. | 5 mg/kg 12 hourly for 2–3 weeks | Haematological toxicity |
| Diarrhoea | Codeine phosphate | Oral | 10–60 mg 4 hourly | Depression of respiration |
| | Loperamide | Oral | 6–16 mg daily | Occasional rashes |
| | Diphenoxylate | Oral | four tabs then two 6 hourly | Dry mouth |
| Gingivitis | Metronidazole | Oral | 200 mg thrice daily | Interaction with alcohol |
| | Choline salicylate | Oral | Topical application | – |
| | Povidone-iodine | Oral | Mouthwash | – |
| Herpes | Acyclovir | Oral | 200–400 mg five times daily | Rash, GIT & CNS symptoms, impaired renal function |
| | | i.v. | 15 mg/kg in 24 hours | |
| HIV | Zidovudine | Oral | 200–300 mg 4 hourly | Haematological toxicity |
| Isosporiasis | Cotrimoxazole | Oral | 480 mg 6 hourly | As for all sulfonamides |
| Toxoplasmosis | Sulfadiazine | Oral | 2–4 g daily | As for all sulfonamides |
| | Pyrimethamine | Oral | 25 mg daily | Marrow suppression, rashes |
| | Clindamycin | Oral | 500 mg four times daily | GIT symptoms |

*continued*

**Table 8.3** *Drugs used in HIV-related disease (continued)*

| Indication | Drug name | Route | Dose range | Important side-effects |
|---|---|---|---|---|
| **Tuberculosis** | Isoniazid | Oral/ i.m | 300–1000 mg twice weekly | Nausea, rash, neuritis, marrow suppression |
| | Rifampicin | Oral | 450–600 mg daily | GIT symptoms, altered liver function — orange/red urine |
| | Streptomycin | i.m. | 500–1000 mg daily | Ototoxicity |
| | Ethambutol | Oral | 15 mg/kg daily | Optic & peripheral neuritis |
| *Pneumocystis carinii* pneumonia (PCP) | Co-trimoxazole | i.v. | 20 mg/kg/ day | Nausea, fever, rash, marrow suppression |
| | Pentamidine | i.v. | 2–4 mg/kg/ day | Hypotension, renal & hepatic failure, hypoglycaemia, marrow suppression |

positive result before the test is carried out. A positive test indicates that the individual is infected with the virus but gives no guide as to prognosis. Seronegativity simply tells one that the individual has not yet converted and does not necessarily mean that he or she is free of the virus or even non-infectious. Unfortunately seropositivity affects the individual, making it difficult for him to obtain life insurance and possibly reducing job prospects. There may be severe psychological upset causing anxiety, guilt or depression with accompanying risk of suicide. It is important that positive results should not be given to a patient on a Friday since counselling services may not be available over the weekend. Seropositivity does not preclude a sex life but partners should observe safer sexual practices.(see Table 8.4).

Once any form of HIV-related illness is diagnosed then counselling is similar to that for cancer except that

**Table 8.4** *Safer sex guidelines*

**No risk**
● Solo masturbation
● Non-genital massage

**Low risk**
● Mutual masturbation
● Dry kissing
● Body rubbing

**Medium risk**
● Wet kissing
● Fellatio (if ejaculation does not occur into the mouth)
● Rimming

**High risk**
● Anal or vaginal sex (without a condom)
● Fisting
● Sharing sex toys and needles
● Any sex act drawing blood

Fellatio = oral intercourse              Rimming = anilingus or insertion of
Fisting = insertion of fist into rectum   tongue into rectum

patients are younger and more prone to feelings of guilt and despair and suicidal attempts are not uncommon. It may be necessary to explore the individual's doubts and worries concerning the course, treatment and outcome of the illness. There will be anxiety about rejection by society or sexual partners, or about the loss of employment, autonomy and self-image. Patients may feel extreme guilt at possibly having infected others especially their loved ones. As with cancer (particularly as the patient becomes very sick) much therapeutic listening is required, with explanation and education about AIDS and stressing the positive aspects of individual cases.

## Symptom control

The majority of patients with HIV-related illness are ambulant and as such are likely to be looked after in the community, where treatment is largely symptomatic and supportive. This is likely to put a heavy burden on primary care as the epidemic increases. In acute episodes admission to hospital may be required, some late cases may need inpatient hospice care but the majority choose to remain at home to die.

As in all palliative care, symptom control depends on identification of cause and the application of the most appropriate treatment. Many AIDS symptoms are due to opportunistic infections or malignancies, which are listed in Table 8.5.

# Respiratory problems

Respiratory symptoms are commonly caused by viral, bacterial, protozoan or fungal infections but may also be caused by pulmonary Kaposi's sarcoma. Some viral infections due to herpes or cytomegalovirus may respond to acyclovir or ganciclovir. Bacterial infection should be treated with the appropriate antibiotic. Infections with atypical forms of mycobacteria respond to antituberculous treatment with combinations of isoniazid, rifampicin, streptomycin and ethambutol. Pneumonia due to *Pneumocystis carinii* is treated with co-trimoxazole 20 mg/kg per day (alternatively pentamidine 4 mg/kg per day may be used). Seventy per cent of patients survive their first episode of *Pneumocystis carinii* pneumonia but may succumb to subsequent attacks. A 2 year survival after the first attack is unusual.

## Gastrointestinal problems

Gastrointestinal symptoms, particularly high-volume diarrhoea, are very common. Many cases are idiopathic but cryptosporidiosis, isospora or microsporidia are among the commoner causes. Bacterial infections include mycobacteria, salmonella and helicobacter. Where possible the cause should be identified and treated, but often this is not possible. No effective treatment exists for cryptosporidiosis but symptomatic relief of diarrhoea due to *Isospora belli* has been reported with trimethoprim-sulfamethoxazole, and with (in America) pyrimethamine-sulfadiazine, and furazolidone. Gastroenteritis due to helicobacter may respond to erythromycin. General

Table 8.5 *Common symptoms in AIDS and their cause*

| System | Symptoms | | | Cause | | |
|---|---|---|---|---|---|---|
| | | Viruses | Bacteria | Protozoa | Fungi | Tumours |
| **Respiratory** | Cough | Cytomegalovirus | Mycobacteria | Pneumocystis carinii | Cryptococcus | Kaposi |
| | Dyspnoea | Herpes simplex | Pneumococcus H. influenzae | | | |
| **Gastrointestinal** | Dysphagia High-volume diarrhoea | Cytomegalovirus Herpes simplex | Mycobacteria Salmonella Helicobacter | Cryptosporidium Isospora belli, Microsporidia | Candida | Kaposi Kaposi |
| **Central nervous system** | Meningitic Encephalitic dementia | Cytomegalovirus Herpes simplex Papovavirus | Mycobacteria | Toxoplasma | Aspergillus Cryptococcus Candida | Lymphoma |
| **Skin** | All skin conditions are worse | Herpes simplex | Staphylococci | | Candida Tinea | Squamous cell |
| **General** | Fever Weight loss Malaise | Consider all types of infection | | | | Any tumour |

symptomatic treatment may require fluid replacement and antidiarrhoeal drugs such as codeine phosphate or loperamide.

Mouth problems due to opportunistic infection consequent on impaired immunity are extremely common and include caries, gingivitis and ulceration of the fauces. Infection may be aphthous, herpetic, fungal or bacterial. Candida is especially common and its presence in the mouth of a young man is highly suggestive of HIV-related illness unless he is using betamethasone aerosols for asthma. Symptomatic relief of herpetic lesions may be obtained with acyclovir, and gingivitis may respond to metronidazole 200 mg thrice daily but eradication of infection is difficult. Symptomatic relief depends on the use of antiseptic mouthwashes and local anaesthetics such as povidone-iodine (Betadine) or choline salicylate (Bonjela).

Tongue lesions are common and hairy leukoplakia (seen as white flat warty projections on the lateral side of the tongue) is pathognomonic of HIV infection. Kaposi's sarcoma, which is most commonly seen on the skin, occurs widely throughout the body, is frequently seen in the mouth and may cause problems, such as dysphagia or obstruction, elsewhere in the gastrointestinal tract.

Dysphagia is commonly due to severe candidal infection, which is often slow to respond to nystatin and may require aggressive treatment with amphotericin or ketoconazole, although the latter may cause further reduction in the number of white cells. Candidiasis may be extremely severe in AIDS, affecting the oesophagus or as a generalised infection with candidaemia.

*Central nervous system problems*

As many as 75% of people with AIDS show postmortem evidence of opportunistic infection of the central nervous system and about one-third of patients with AIDS develop a subacute encephalitis caused by HIV. In mild cases there may be forgetfulness and loss of concentration with lethargy and loss of motor function; more severe cases show dementia. Often in people with AIDs there may be several different HIV-related diseases in any one individual and HIV encephalopathy may coexist with opportunistic infection or tumours.

Meningitis may occur in AIDS due to *Cryptococcus neoformans*. It is less florid in its symptomatology than acute bacterial meningitis but may resemble tuberculous meningitis. It presents with malaise and fever, headache with nausea and vomiting and there may be photophobia and neck stiffness. Space-occupying lesions may be caused by opportunistic infection such as toxoplasmosis, or abscesses caused by mycobacteria or candida. Other neurological manifestations of AIDS occur as progressive multifocal leucoencephalopathy (a form of demyelinating disease) retinitis and peripheral neuropathy.

Treatment of neurological disease depends on treating the opportunistic infection where possible. Systemic fungal infection may respond to amphotericin, atypical mycobacteria respond to standard antituberculous therapy and toxoplasmosis requires long-term treatment with sulfonamides, clindamycin and pyrimethamine.

*Skin conditions*

Almost all skin conditions become more florid in the presence of immunosuppression. All infective skin conditions, viral, bacterial or fungal, are particularly severe and may require energetic treatment with topical acyclovir, antibiotic or antifungal cream or ointment.

*Tumours*

The commonest tumour is Kaposi's sarcoma. Individual lesions may occur anywhere but are most commonly seen in the skin or mouth. They are multifocal and pigmented, often purplish or brown and arise from vascular endothelium. Starting as a tiny skin blemish they rapidly develop and may be widespread. There is no specific treatment but radiotherapy may have useful cosmetic effect on visible lesions.

Other malignant tumours include lymphoma and some forms of squamous cell cancer. Response to radiotherapy is poor and treatment is largely symptomatic.

## General symptoms

General symptoms such as depression, fever, malaise, weakness and anorexia occur frequently in HIV-related disease; there is no specific treatment and the same principles apply to AIDS as to the palliative care of cancer.

Sometimes patients in the late stages of AIDS may wish to go home to die. This may result in the family doctor and community services being faced with enormously complicated problems for which they may have had little training. In some parts of Britain hospice home care teams are building up considerable expertise in this aspect of palliative care and may be able to offer a great deal of help.

CHAPTER 9

# Help from the hospice

THE word hospice derives from the latin *hospitium*: a stranger or guest. From this stem a number of words arise such as host, hospitable, hospital and hospice. Originally a hospice was a place of entertainment for strangers where a host (one who entertains strangers) would be hospitable (kind to strangers). Originally the word hospital had nothing to do with the sick but was a place for receiving pilgrims or a charitable institution for the elderly, infirm or orphaned. The author's somewhat Victorian father used to refer to his local pub as a 'hospice'; it is perhaps a pity that this image is not a commoner one.

The history of the hospice movement started with charitable monastic institutions set up by religious orders. St Luke's Hospital for the Incurable, the first modern hospice, was founded in London in 1893, followed by St Joseph's in 1905. The foundation of St Christopher's in 1967 established high standards of care and research in hospice medicine. Now there are over a hundred hospices in Britain and many in North America and Australasia.

Though there is considerable variation between individual hospices in Britain they generally serve three main functions:

- care of patients in their own homes by means of advisory home care teams;
- provision of day care facilities for ambulant patients;

- admission facilities for symptom control, respite care or the continuing care of patients who for various reasons cannot be managed in their own homes or appropriate institutions.

Hospices offer holistic care for patients' physical, psychological, social and spiritual needs. It follows that their staffing must cater for all these aspects of care. There is usually a medical director, who is often backed up by a senior house officer and often with support from local general practitioners. A few hospices now have senior registrars training for future consultancy. In addition a number of universities have academic posts in palliative care funded by the Cancer Relief Macmillan Fund.

Nursing is of paramount importance and the levels of nursing staff are similar to those found in intensive care units. Nurses undergo special courses of training in the care of patients with advanced cancer. Although this often involves highly skilled practical nursing there is also a need for great communication skills.

Hospices often have a foundation based on religion or even a single Christian denomination but they have access to spiritual advisers from other denominations and most religions. While this is very important it sometimes creates the false impression that patients need to be of a given creed. One sometimes hears a patient say 'I am not religious so I cannot go to a hospice.' Needless to say this is totally wrong and patients may need reassurance about this. Social aspects of care are extremely important and expert social workers guide patients through the complexity of regulations governing benefits. They are also often involved in counselling and in bereavement follow-up.

Running hospices, which generally receive only minimal financial support from the National Health Service, is an extremely complex business requiring full-time administrative staff. Domestic staff provide excellent catering that is quite different from traditional hospital food. In all these fields professional staff are supported by huge numbers of specially trained volunteers who help to reduce the institutional flavour of a hospice to an absolute minimum.

## Work of a hospice

This varies somewhat between hospices. All hospices care for patients with cancer and most will also take on a small proportion of patients with chronic non-cancerous disease, particularly neurological disease such as multiple sclerosis or motor neurone disease. Increasingly hospices are being asked to accept the care of people with AIDS. Policy varies with regard to AIDS and local advice should be sought. Equally some hospices such as the London Lighthouse cater exclusively for AIDS.

There are now hospices throughout the British Isles and there is an excellent and frequently updated directory of hospices available from St Christopher's Hospice.[1] The Hospice Information Service in London can provide further information about location of the nearest hospice and the facilities provided.[2] Table 9.1 depicts a single small hospice's annual workload, which may help to correct misconceptions about its function.

## Referrals

In a typical British hospice two-thirds of referrals come from general practitioners, another tenth from primary care nurses and about one-fifth from hospitals. Other sources of referral include district nurses or social workers in the community and occasionally from patients or their relatives. In some areas there may be home care teams working from hospitals or the community, who, though not based in a hospice, may refer to nearby hospices. An important feature of referral is that permission of the patient's general practitioner is always sought before acceptance of a referral from any other source. Failure to do this may lead to duplication of effort or communication difficulties. It is not the function of

**Table 9.1** *Annual workload of a nineteen bed hospice*

| Referrals | *Source of referral* | *Number* | % |
|---|---|---|---|
| | G.P. | 309 | 64.1 |
| | Hospital | 102 | 21.2 |
| | District nurse | 46 | 9.5 |
| | Social worker | 2 | 0.4 |
| | Patient | 1 | 0.2 |
| | Relative of patient | 3 | 0.6 |
| | Nearby home | 19 | 4.0 |
| | Total | 482 | 100 |
| **Total workload** | | *Number* | % |
| ● New referrals | | 482 | |
| ● Patients visited by home care team: | | | |
| | mean no. per month | 155 | |
| | range | 129–193 | |
| ● Total visits by home care team | | 2193 | |
| ● Admissions to hospice: | | | |
| | new | 196 | |
| | readmissions | 61 | |
| | Total | 257 | |
| ● Live discharges | | 105 | 40.8 |
| ● Deaths: | | | |
| | in hospice | 147 | 37.1 |
| | at home | 174 | 43.9 |
| | in hospital | 75 | 19.0 |
| | Total (some patients from previous year) | 396 | |
| ● Attending day centre | | 126 | |
| ● Total attendances at day centre | | 1324 | |

*Source:* F.M. Hull & J.H. Taylor, 'Quality and Quantity in Palliative Care', *Update* 40, 1990, pp. 269–74.

the hospice to take over the work of primary care but to supplement and augment it.

Certain information is obviously essential on referring patients to the hospice and for this reason most hospices provide referral forms requesting details of diagnosis, prognosis, the patient's state of knowledge of the illness and medication.

Unfortunately the laity have a mistaken image of hospices, which is only slowly being corrected. A hospice is often seen as a place of death, with the result that frequently people refuse to accept the advantages of hospice care. Many patients attend hospice facilities for several years and learn how to live with cancer thus giving meaning to the slogan that hospices 'add life to years rather than years to life'. Thus referral early in the natural history of cancer is important; equally there is no point whatsoever in the transfer of a moribund patient except in cases of extreme carer's distress.

Most referrals are looked after by the primary care teams based on general practices. The hospice home care team supports the primary care team with assistance from their medical director, who will visit the patients at the request of the general practitioner or the home care sister with the general practitioner's approval. It is generally accepted that a majority of patients wish to die at home and the medical and nursing advice of the hospice home care team may be invaluable in making this possible. As a general rule the home care team is advisory without offering practical nursing or medical skills but it does have access to special nursing equipment and syringe drivers, which may make home care possible. Through the hospice social worker there may be access to special funds to help with the purchase of extra help, equipment or holidays.

Table 9.1 showed that out of 482 referrals in a year at a small hospice there were only some 257 admissions, of which many were readmissions.[1] Many referrals are cared for at home throughout the course of their illness and may never be admitted to the hospice at all.

Patients who are well enough attend the day care centre for one or more days per week. In the day centre they have the opportunity to discuss their progress with medical and nursing staff and, more importantly, with each other. The day centre provides peer-group support, recreational and social functions and facilities for dressings, checking medication, bathing and hairdressing. This is often much appreciated by patients, who look forward to their visit as a weekly treat. Often the hospice will provide entertainment in the form of concerts, parties and outings. Birthdays call for special cakes and celebrations and lunch is often preceded with a glass of a favourite drink from the bar. Patients have been known to attend the day centre for many years and the atmosphere of friendship can be quite remarkable. For these people especially the hospice is about living, not about dying.

It often comes as a surprise to people with little experience of hospices that two-fifths of admissions are discharged home alive. About equal numbers of patients die at home as in the hospice and a further fifth die in hospital. When there are particular problems such as with pain, vomiting or confusion, patients may be admitted for symptom control. Once the symptom is no longer a problem the patient may return home to be cared for by the general practitioner and community nurse backed up by the hospice home care team. Another reason for admission is to provide respite for carers at home to allow them to take a holiday. Lastly patients may be admitted for continuing care during the last stages of illness for medical or social reasons. Many of our patients come in near the end of their lives simply because there is inadequate support at home. Many patients are elderly and cared for by a spouse of the same age group, who may not be able to cope with the problem because of their own infirmity. Such patients are in marked contrast to people with AIDS, who are much younger and with carers of their own age.

Though hospices are repositories of great caring skills it is important to realise that there is nothing that is done in a hospice that cannot also be done at home or even in a hospital ward. Unfortunately this often does not happen.

## CHAPTER 10

# Alternative care

ALTERNATIVE or complementary medicine has little or no place in the curative treatment of cancer. However, once the decision to abandon pursuit of cure and adopt palliative care then it has a great deal to offer. If nothing else complementary methods, by making the patient *feel* better even in the absence of evidence of real improvement, enhance the cancer sufferer's quality of life. But there is much more to complementary medicine than just subjective improvement.

There are scores of different complementary therapies each with their exponents and devotees. It is not the purpose of this book to describe them because details are available elsewhere (for example Hull, Ellis & Sargent — see 'Further reading' for Chapters 3–6). Rather it is useful to offer some explanation of how complementary care may help patients.

Undoubtedly more and more people consult practitioners of complementary medicine. In Britain alone more than a million people consult some 30 000 practitioners of complementary medicine a year. In America and Australasia the figures are even higher. Studies in Belgium suggest that the popularity of complementary medicine is related to the greater amount of time offered to patients by its practitioners compared with conventional doctors. But how can more time produce beneficial effect in conjunction with what are often quite bizarre methods of treatment?

To answer this question it is necessary to approach it at a tangent by considering a number of strange and, until recently, unexplained observations. If one were to match a hundred recently bereaved people by age and sex with a non-bereaved group and study their mortality rates there would be an excess of deaths in the bereaved group. If suicide (which might be directly related to bereavement) were excluded then the excess mortality would be caused by myocardial infarcts, infections, particularly pneumonia, and cancer.

Not only is there a preponderance of cancer deaths among the bereaved but patients commonly attribute the onset of their cancer to some form of shock. Certainly talking to patients in hospices it is surprising how often this seemingly nonsensical assertion is made. Yet another puzzle is offered by patients who survive severe malignancies against all medical expectation and this contrasts with patients who 'turn their faces to the wall' and die unexpectedly quickly from cancer. Such cases bring to mind the wasting condition that is recorded among primitive peoples subjected to the 'evil eye' 'voodoo' or, in Aboriginals, 'the pointing of the bone'.

In fact all these bizarre observations are linked. Our understanding of this linkage has developed from knowledge derived from, among other sources, AIDS. Derangement of the function of the immune system sheds light on the way it protects against cancer. At any one time in most people there are potentially malignant cells, but we do not all get cancer because the cells of the immune system identify these aberrant cells as being foreign and destroy them. In AIDS a deficiency of T4 cells interferes with this defence mechanism and either unusual infections or certain types of cancer may result. It can be shown that the numbers of T4 cells is depleted following adverse life situations such as bereavement, loss or other severe stress. Even examinations may produce this result — lymphocyte counts have been shown to fall in medical students before major exams. It is probable that a similar impairment of the immune system occurs in cases of 'evil eye'.

This offers an explanation for patients developing, or rather failing to prevent, the onset of cancer, after adverse life situations. It may also help to explain why a patient survives or even apparently recovers from widespread cancer — the complex balance between the emotional state and the immune system adjusts and the cancer is controlled. If adverse circumstances depress the immune system then it seems logical that a patient who can maintain a high quality of life may actually boost his or her ability to resist the disease.

The idea of a close relationship between brain, hormones, neurotransmitters and immunity is now sometimes referred to as the 'psychoneuro-endocrineimmune system'. This concept puts a new complexion on palliative care that aims to improve the quality of life rather than its quantity. This is sometimes referred to as adding life to years rather than years to life. The interesting point is that improving quality of life may also improve its quantity. If this is so, then any form of complementary care, however bizarre it may seem, is worth trying provided it does not involve the patient in physical, psychological, social or spiritual hardship. Even more importantly this concept of balance between mind and body stresses the need for the very best communication, listening, understanding and empathy with the patient undergoing palliative care of AIDS or cancer.

CHAPTER 11

# Death, dying and bereavement

MEDICAL and lay voices are increasingly raised in protest at insensitive behaviour of doctors towards dying patients and their relatives. This is particularly true of junior doctors who have suddenly made the metamorphosis from medical student to having to care for extremely ill people, being exposed to dying patients and their relatives when stressed by fatigue and the anxiety of responsibility. Though they may have little experience of death and less teaching about it, they are suddenly regarded by lay people as being experts in death. These obvious deficiencies prompted a study of the experience of and attitudes towards death and dying among students at Birmingham Medical School.

In 1900 death was a frequent experience, many families lost children and young adults from infection and trauma. Death occurred at home and society both accepted and adapted to it. A young man or woman of twenty would be most unlikely to have no experience of death and some would have been involved in the loss of many close relatives including siblings. Nowadays things are different; at the end of the twentieth century death has become sanitised, it occurs out of sight in institutions and the majority of people rarely see dead bodies. Society as a whole has little experience of death and, when suddenly faced with it in themselves or their close relatives, turn to doctors as supposed experts. But newly qualified doctors have almost as little experience themselves; no wonder problems arise.

Ahmedzai[1] reported the resident's viewpoint on dying in hospital in 1982, when 64% of junior house officers thought they had received inadequate teaching in terminal care. They thought nursing staff much more helpful than senior medical staff with regard to both medical and psychological aspects of terminal care and that there was need for more teaching on how to cope with the psychological problems of dying patients. Cox[2] writing the reflections of a medical student on care of the dying in 1987 described the need for medical students to spend more time with and have more teaching about the dying. This is particularly true of cancer patients towards whom medical students often hold negative attitudes.

There are deficiencies in many communication skills, especially in informing patients of bad news; this deficiency even worsens with passage through medical school. That this is allowed to happen despite the knowledge that the majority of patients wish to know the truth about diagnosis and prognosis is a poor reflection of medical teaching at the end of the twentieth century. Even though many medical schools now teach about the breaking of bad news and that students perceive breaking bad news as an important part of the doctor's task they are confused, uncertain and insecure about it and clearly demand help and guidance in what they see as a very difficult area.

A questionnaire, adapted from a similar document used by Stedeford and Twycross[3] in teaching palliative care at Oxford was distributed to students at Birmingham Medical School in their first and third clinical years.[4] The questionnaire was answered by 119 third-year and 143 final-year students. One-quarter recorded that the death of a pet was their first lasting impression of death but the majority (58%) mentioned deaths of relatives or acquaintances. Sixteen per cent of students had no experience of death within the family. Where family deaths had occurred these were mostly among grandparents. Twenty-seven deaths of the parental generation were mentioned, thirteen among parents themselves. Only two students mentioned the death of a sibling. The deaths were not only distant by kinship but also temporally, with 168 deaths occurring more than 2 years previously.

Males, more accident prone, were more likely to have experience of peer-group death than were female students. It is, however, surprising that more than two-fifths of students have experience of death within their peer groups. It is again noticeable how frequently violent death is mentioned. At least one-third of all students have never been to a funeral of someone they know well and less than a third of students had seen or touched a dead body before reaching the medical school. During the clinical years the number of students who have talked to people who knew that they were dying rose from less than a third to just over half. That is to say that only about one-fifth of students increased this aspect of their experience of death and dying during their clinical years, and of these some came in contact with death in their social lives rather than their work.

When posed the question 'what would you want to be told if you had cancer and only 6 months to live?', the majority either wanted to know everything about the disease (76%) or wanted information about the quality of life that they might expect (18%). There is no reason to believe that these findings are peculiar to Birmingham. Clearly students become doctors with little formal teaching about death and dying. Such experience as they do acquire is more likely to have come before entry to the medical school or in their social lives. This is bound to have a bearing on their communication skills as young doctors when they are thrown in at the deep end of house jobs.

The above findings indicate the need for special teaching about death and dying. It is essential that such teaching should occur at times of special difficulty for students: just before human dissection, immediately prior to clinical studies, and as late in the course as possible so that they are prepared for dealing with death among their patients as house officers. There is also a need for special counselling services within medical schools to help students adjust to their own personal traumas whether these result from work or from deaths among their families or friends. The student who cannot come to terms with his or her own experience of death is not likely to be able to help patients or their relatives later in professional life. That there is a need for increased teaching with regard to the care of people with advanced and incurable disease is exemplified by two comments written by students after a course in palliative care at Birmingham.

> I dreaded coming to the hospice and having to talk to people about dying but realise there is nothing to worry about. I feel it's been a very useful time and very important to improve my attitude towards death and dying. I've enjoyed this afternoon so much that I could even consider working in palliative care . . . something I wouldn't have dreamt of before.

> It seems a shame that our medical school can only find a day and a half to give teaching of this sort when it can find in excess of 30 weeks of medicine and surgery. Isn't there something wrong somewhere?

Balfour Mount,[5] Canada's doyen of palliative care, stresses the importance of acceptance of death, not as weakness but as the antithesis of denial. He suggests a number of important considerations that influence such acceptance including the following:

- Knowledge of death runs through life influencing everything we do, think and believe.
- Many changes in twentieth century society have severely undermined our ability to deal with death.
- In consequence, care of the seriously ill and dying has suffered.
- So have our own lives.

- Awareness of issues surrounding death and dying influences our own professional and personal lives.
- A patient's experience of his or her illness is shaped by his or her self-perception and it is only through understanding of this perception that a carer can understand the way the patient feels.
- We bring to our professional roles as care givers our feelings about our own mortality and therefore we can only help others if we have come to understand and accept that mortality.

Many of these considerations come with maturity; it may be difficult for young men and women working as junior doctors to appreciate these attitudes to death and dying. Teaching by discussion and thinking oneself into the situation of patients will help to foster appreciation of how it feels to be dying.

In this context Balfour Mount[5] quotes Schweitzer: 'it is our duty to remember at all times and anew that medicine is not only a science but also the art of letting our own individuality interact with the individuality of the patient'.

Mount also has suggestions about the management of death:

- The family should be present if possible, even though the experience of death may be traumatic at the time, the ability to see it happen, to say goodbye and to lessen the feeling of guilt at absence more than compensates.
- Family members should see the body after death again; this is a time for goodbyes and acceptance, which will lessen grieving later.
- Children have fewer problems with death than adults imagine and it often helps both them and the other relatives if they are involved with the death.
- Give everybody plenty of time.
- When death occurs in hospital get the family to collect and pack up the person's belongings because

that is much more personal than being handed a plastic bag of junk.

- Say a prayer at the death or over the body in the presence of the family because this formalises the business of death. Strangely some of the most unlikely people who seem offhand at the time later say how much they valued this.
- Touch the body and facilitate touching by the relatives.
- Arrange an autopsy: relatives want to know what happened; it concretises the loss and deals with questions.
- After death go to the funeral. Why is it we don't go? Is it because this is a reminder of failure? Are we callous or afraid of death? We don't go because we don't know that it is important since it allows a review of the case, increases the significance of the dead person, it respects the family and it respects one's own feelings.

## Bereavement

Kübler-Ross in her seminal book *On Death and Dying* describes stages of the bereavement reaction as follows: denial, isolation and searching; anger; depression; acceptance.

It is important to realise that patients with advanced cancer are themselves undergoing bereavement in that they too are shortly to be deprived of life, their loved ones and all their treasured possessions. They too go through the same stages in the process of coming to terms with impending death but here Kübler-Ross adds the stage of bargaining as a third stage between those of anger and depression. Though these stages can often be clearly distinguished they may run together or overlap. A peculiar but quite common feature of grief is hallucination. This may occur in any bereavement but is commoner between spouses particularly after long and successful marriage.

Occasionally an abnormal bereavement pattern may develop with severe and pathological exaggeration of any of its stages. Denial can lead to withdrawal from reality. Anger may be so extreme as to develop into vendetta but these behaviour patterns are fortunately rare. A much commoner abnormal grief reaction leads to severe depression, with classical early morning waking, feelings of worthlessness and suicidal thoughts. The risk of pathological grief is higher with low social class, male gender and youth. Religious activity and personality show only weak correlations with severe bereavement reactions but the duration and nature of the terminal illness, especially if it were violent or suicidal death, may be indicators of abnormal grief. The state of the marital relationship is also important especially where the remaining spouse had felt dependent on or ambivalent towards the dead person.

*Morbidity of bereavement*

Bereavement has a substantial mortality and morbidity. For centuries it has been observed that death rates are higher among the bereaved than the non-bereaved. Recent work has shown that this effect may be produced as a result of altered catecholamine metabolism in the brain, which may lead to altered behaviour patterns and abnormal stress reactions. Altered catecholamine metabolism may have a direct effect on the cardiovascular system leading to raised blood pressure, heart failure and myocardial infarction. But there is also evidence of changes in the immune system especially on T-lymphocyte function in bereavement and allied emotional states (see Chapter 10).

*Management of bereavement*

The management of bereavement depends more on listening than anything else and as such is very time consuming. Perhaps this is the reason that it is often neglected. There may be lingering doubts in the carer's mind that more could have been done. Such doubt is only too human after a death and it may help to explore this with the relatives. Follow up should be arranged, where possible by the doctor but often this is impractical, when it should be carried out by nursing or social work staff.

In cases where anger or other emotional turmoil smoulders discussion may do much to allow ventilation of pent-up feelings. In many cases the carer has no other function than to listen to the chronicle of the deceased's last illness and hours. This is very comforting to those who are left behind who may be able, through talking, to assuage their own conflicting feelings of sadness, anger or guilt about the death. As John Donne reminds us 'No man is an island, entire of itself . . . Any man's death diminishes me, because I am involved in Mankind; And therefore never send to know for whom the bell tolls; it tolls for thee'. So one must be aware of the effect of death on a ward, street or locality. When there is a cluster of deaths, a distressing death or of some special, or very young patient, this has its effect on carers. It may be necessary to spend time discussing the case to allow emotional adjustment. Whole sections of the population may undergo mass grief reactions especially after the presence of multiple deaths or disasters such as the Lockerbie air crash. Such circumstances require the services of specially trained counsellors with experience of disaster care.

## CHAPTER 12

# Breaking bad news

B REAKING bad news is an inevitable part of the doctor's role. Though every occasion is different there are some basic rules that, if they do not make it easier, perhaps render it less difficult.

First it is important to realise that there are three forms of communication: speech, figurative speech and dreams, and non-verbal communication. Eighty per cent of our communication is non-verbal and the rest variously distributed between direct and figurative speech. Much of our non-verbal communication is involuntary and it reflects our most hidden feelings. But this form of communication can be controlled and used to help and support the recipient of bad news. Actors train themselves to express their emotions through non-verbal communication and sometimes the hidden emotion is at total variance from the emotional content of their spoken words. This illustrates how spoken and non-verbal communication may contradict each other and it also shows how the non-verbal can be controlled. Doctors must be aware of the congruence or non-congruence of non-verbal communication especially when talking to people in distress.

## Advice to those faced with breaking bad news

There are many barriers to communication. Some may be in the physical environment: noise, bustle, lack of privacy.

These are the easiest to control. Some may be in the receiver or transmitter of information, which will be more difficult. Before attempting to break bad news it is important that you try to identify the major barriers so that they can be anticipated and overcome.

## Physical barriers

It is important that there is quiet and privacy. It is important that communication is seen to be unhurried, this may be one of the most difficult impressions to give in the busy routine of a house officer, nevertheless this is one of the doctor's most important functions and certainly the one by which you will be judged. Recipients of bad news may be the patient or relatives; so let us borrow a term from other disciplines and call them clients. The client should be in a warm quiet room apart from the general hubbub of the hospital. If possible the room should be homely, not the stark side office of a busy hospital ward. The client should be seated comfortably. Take someone else with you, circumstances will dictate who that should be but it will usually be a nurse. It may be that if you are of different gender from the client then the third person should be the same as the client. This may be important, for example in informing a woman of the diagnosis of breast or cervical cancer when it may help her to have another woman present. There are several reasons for a third person. Sometimes it is necessary to have a means of getting messages out of the room without leaving the client alone. In the often emotionally charged atmosphere it may be important for someone else to hear what is said since the words and content may be forgotten or not taken in by the client. Lastly it enables you to leave, as may be demanded by other calls on medical time, without leaving the client alone. If you are called away by pressure of work this must be accompanied by apology and information should be passed to nursing staff that there is now only one person with the client.

*Barriers in the client*

Clients may be already anticipating bad news or it may be completely unexpected. Where news is not unexpected reaction may be denial or anger. Whatever the reaction in the client he or she must be given time and hearing. Denial is always difficult to cope with since it is a refusal to accept the message that has to be delivered; all one can do is to repeat it and try again another time. Anger is easier but often dealt with badly. It is human nature to seek some source of blame; this, however unjustly, may be the giver of the news. This is nothing new — the Greeks used to execute the bearers of bad news! Anger may be directed at the doctors, sometimes with reason, more often just because they are available. In their grief, clients may want to grumble at God for the distress, but the doctor is right there! Sometimes the client's anger is directed at herself or himself for real or imagined omissions. Such guilt may be devastating and requires much patience and listening.

Where the bad news is not expected there will usually be shock, disbelief and total non-acceptance . . . 'but I saw him only this morning . . .'. Again this will need much time and patience on the part of the doctor. This will involve telling the client as much as may be known about the events that led to death or broad details of the cause of death or injury. We tend to seek comfort for ourselves in platitudes such as 'at least he knew nothing about it', which may help the client too.

Sometimes reactions are unexpected even involving a black form of humour. Under such circumstances it may be difficult not to respond inappropriately. A patient of mine whose husband died in the middle of a meal in an expensive restaurant complained that he had not paid the bill!

*Barriers in the doctor*

The commonest barriers are fear, shame, guilt, anger, sadness and our impotence at the event. The greatest limiting factor is often time. It is essential that time be made available; the commonest complaint is that the doctor did not care. Often he or she cared a great deal but was too rushed or embarrassed to show it. Fear is a barrier because one can imagine oneself in the position of the client and feel that one could not cope. Shame may be felt because of a sense of injustice and waste. This may be particularly keen when a young person is killed in an accident. Guilt may be felt because of self-perceived inadequacy ... 'if only I had known how to...'. Anger, like that of the client, may be at Fate, or God, for allowing this to happen. In aggression or war this may be directed at the enemy with vows of vengeance.

Sadness may be overwhelming and there is little escape from it. Perhaps, as doctors, we try too hard to suppress our sadness at some of the events we witness. It cannot harm us to express our own grief and our clients will respect us all the more for it. Perhaps the most confusing emotion is that of impotence, which, though compounded of all the other emotions, can be the most difficult to deal with. The helplessness felt, for example, when standing with an unbelieving mother by the cot in which an apparently normal child has died, has to be experienced to be understood. It combines anger and futility, which may render one helpless to help. The only way one can help is by sharing one's grief.

*How it may be done*

Of course there is no single answer; each time it is different but there are some guidelines. Firstly recognise the barriers and try to circumvent them. Where this is impossible it will help to see them clearly and possibly to share them with the client. Be in command of both the facts and your own emotions. Make sure there is quiet and comfort and that you have someone to help you. See that the client is seated and sit yourself so that you are near to that person. You will need to judge, by being sensitive to the client's non-verbal communication, the degree of closeness. Some people feel threatened by invasion of their personal space, others need the reassurance of human proximity and touch. Speak slowly and clearly, using simple words, for even the most intelligent, when afflicted with grief, may not hear or may misunderstand. Stop frequently to let your message be digested. If necessary ask if the client understands. As soon as the client speaks stop and listen intently watching for non-verbal cues.

Your own non-verbal communication is vitally important. Sit leaning forward in attention so that the client feels that you are concentrating on him or her to the exclusion of everything else. Keep your eyes at the level of the client's eyes making contact as much as you can. Keep still. There is no shame in weeping; better people than you have done it before. That does not mean collapsing in a tearstained wreck but, as Balfour Mount puts it, 'acceptance not as weakness but as the antithesis of denial'.[1] The knowledge that you suffer too may make the client's ordeal bearable. Sometimes roles are reversed and the client consoles the doctor. There is nothing wrong with that, for the client in giving may receive strength.

Be prepared to touch the client if that seems appropriate. A supportive hand on shoulder or even an arm round a distressed person may be consoling and a demonstration of care. Touch is often difficult in British culture. A survey among British and Dutch medical students[2] showed that while it was proper to console an injured dog by patting it or soothe a child by hugging it, it was a different matter when dealing with an adult human devastated by disaster. Touch may be the most appropriate form of consolation. It may take the form of an arm round a shoulder, hand-holding or even an embrace.

In an attempt to help teach about breaking bad news a videotape of this name has been made in conjunction with Birmingham University, Warwickshire Police and a theological college.[3]

In some cases it may be helpful to refer the client to appropriate helping agencies or support groups (see Appendix 1).

# Special problems of breaking bad news

*Identification*

Sometimes, particularly after accidental death, there may be a need for identification of a body. Some bodies are badly disfigured. Obviously the ordeal must be made as easy as possible by hiding the worst of the trauma. It is well to assume that most people have never seen a dead body, let alone someone dear to them. The doctor should see the body before showing it to relatives and so be in a position to warn about its appearance. It may help to warn that the body will be pale but otherwise the appearance will be of sleep with eyes open. Where possible the surroundings of identification should be as un-clinical as possible, preferably with the body in a normal bed. The client should be given space and time, with the attendant being sensitive to the need for solitude or company. Needs are different for everyone and grief is individual; sometimes the client may wish to touch, hold or kiss the body and this may prove of great solace later. The client may wish to be alone, if so the attendant should remain close by ready to help if necessary. Afterwards there will be a need for the client to sit down and perhaps speak about the dead person and his or her feelings about that person. The traditional cup of tea gives everyone something to do.

*Consent to postmortem*

Sometimes it may be necessary to obtain consent for postmortem examination. Where death has been violent, or of unknown cause, there may be a statutory need for autopsy. This will need to be explained but is usually accepted since the need is well known. Where additional examination of the body is needed for medical purposes things may be more difficult. Relatives may regard the request for a postmortem examination as further disfigurement purely for medical purposes. It is necessary to be prepared with good reasons for a request for autopsy. Where the doctors are well known to the client and trusted by them the suggestion that the death may help to help others with the same problem may be consoling for relatives.

### Consent to organ donation

This can be very difficult since it often occurs after young traumatic deaths when time is at a premium. Obviously it is greatly helped by the carrying of donor cards. It may help to stress that even in death the person may be able to help fellow human beings.

The guiding principle in all this must be to take time, listen, watch and be aware of all the verbal and non-verbal cues that are offered.

It is never easy, even after a lifetime in medicine.

# Bibliography

## Preface

*References*

1   F. M. Hull, 'Palliative Care: Introductory Editorial', *Journal of Clinical Pharmacy and Therapeutics* 15, 1990, pp. 301–2.

2   F. M. Hull, 'The Management of Pain in Advanced Cancer', *Journal of Clinical Pharmacy and Therapeutics* 15, 1990, pp. 303–6.

3   F. M. Hull, 'Palliative Care: Gastrointestinal Symptoms I', *Journal of Clinical Pharmacy and Therapeutics* 15, 1990, pp. 307–11.

4   F. M. Hull, 'Palliative Care: Gastrointestinal Symptoms II'. *Journal of Clinical Pharmacy and Therapeutics* 15, 1990, pp. 381–5.

5   F. M. Hull, 'Palliative Care: Physical Symptoms I, Respiratory and Central Nervous System', *Journal of Clinical Pharmacy and Therapeutics* 15, 1990, pp. 387–92.

6   F. M. Hull, 'Palliative Care: Physical Symptoms II', *Journal of Clinical Pharmacy and Therapeutics* 15, 1990, pp. 463–7.

7   F. M. Hull, 'Palliative Care: Psychological Problems, *Journal of Clinical Pharmacy and Therapeutics* 15, 1990, pp. 469–73.

## Chapter 2

*References*

[1] R. G. Twycross and S. A. Lack, *Symptom Control in Far Advanced Cancer: Pain Relief*, Pitman Publishing, London, 1983.

[2] B. M. Mount, personal communication.

[3] A. Dejgard, P. Petersen and J. Kastrup, *Lancet* i, 1988, pp. 9–11.

*Further reading*

Hull, F. M. unpublished report to 'Help the Hospices' following a fellowship at Memorial Sloane Kettering Cancer Center, New York, April, 1990.
Saunders, C., *The Management of Terminal Illness*, London Hospital Medical Publications, London, 1967.

## Chapters 3–6

*Reference*

[1] D. G. Grahame-Smith and J. K. Aronson, *The Oxford Textbook of Clinical Pharmacology and Drug Therapy*, Oxford University Press, Oxford 1984.

*Further reading*

Doyle, D., *Domiciliary Terminal Care*, Churchill Livingstone, Edinburgh, 1987.

Hanratty, J. F., *Palliative Care of the Terminally Ill*, Radcliffe Medical Press, Oxford, 1989.

Hull, R., Ellis, M. and Sargent, V., *Teamwork in Palliative Care*, Radcliffe Medical Press, Oxford, 1989.

Regnard, C. F. B. and Tempest, S., *A Guide to Symptom relief in Advanced Cancer* (3rd edn), Haigh & Hochland Ltd, Manchester, 1992.

Spilling, R. (ed.), *Terminal Care at Home*, Oxford Medical Publications, Oxford, 1986.

## Chapter 7

*Reference*
[1]  F. M. Hull, 'The Management of Depression', in *Treatment in General Practice,* Kluwer publishing, Brentford, 1988, Section 3.7.

## Chapter 8

*References*
[1]  Communicable Disease Surveillance Centre 1993, *Communicable Disease Report,* 3 (43), 197–200.
[2]  M. W. Adler, personal communication (lecture 5/3/91).

*Further reading*
Adler, M. W. (ed.), 'ABC of AIDS', *British Medical Journal,* London. 1987.

Adler, M. W. (ed.), *Disease in the Homosexual Male,* Springer–Verlag, London, 1988.

Expert Advisory Group on AIDS, *Guidance for Clinical Health Care Workers: Protection Against Infection with HIV and Hepatitis Viruses,* Her Majesty's Stationery Office, London. 1990.

Greenspan, D., Pindborg, J. J., Greenspan, J. S. and Schidt, M., *AIDS and the Dental Team,* Munksgard, Copenhagen, 1986.

Hull, R. *Infective Disease in Primary Care,* Chapman and Hall, London, 1987.

Shilts, R., *And the Band Played On,* Penguin, Harmondsworth, 1987.

Wells, N., *The AIDS Virus, Forecasting its Impact,* Office of Health Economics, London, 1987.

## Chapter 9

*References*
[1]  F. M. Hull and J. H. Taylor, 'Quality and Quantity in Palliative Care', *Update* 40, 1990, pp. 269–74.
[2]  Hospice Information Service, 51/53 Lawrie Park Road, Sydenham SE26 6DZ.

*Further reading*

Saunders, C., 'Death, Dying and the Hospice Movement', in J. Walton, B. Beeson and R. Bodley Scott, *The Oxford Companion to Medicine,* Oxford University Press, Oxford, 1986.

## Chapter 10

*Further reading*

Kasl, S. V., Evans, A. S. and Neidermam, J. C., 'Psychosocial Risk Factors in the Development of Infectious Mononucleosis', *Psychosomatic Medicine* 41, 1979, pp. 445–6.

Kennedy, S., Kiecolt-Glaser, J. K. and Glaser, R., 'Immunological Consequences of Acute and Chronic Stressors: Mediating Role of Interpersonal Relationships', *British Journal of Medical Psychology* 61, 1988, pp. 77–85.

Kiecolt-Glaser, J. K., Garner, W., Speicher, C., Penn, G. M., Holliday, J. and Glaser, R., 'Psychosocial Modifiers of Immunocompetence in Medical Students', *Psychosomatic Medicine* 46, 1984, pp. 7–14.

Lewith, G. T. and Kenyon, J. N., 'Physiological and Psychological Explanations for the Mechanism of Acupuncture as a Treatment for Chronic Pain', *Social Science and Medicine* 19, 1984, pp. 1367–78.

Ornstein, R. and Sobel, D., *The Healing Brain: a Radical New Approach to Health Care*, Macmillan, London, 1988.

Osterweis, M., Solomon, F. and Green, M. (eds), *Bereavement: Reactions, Consequences and Care,* National Academy Press, Washington, 1984, pp. 157–70.

Stroebe, W. and Stroebe, M. S., *Bereavement and Health*, Cambridge University Press, Cambridge, 1987.

## Chapter 11

*References*

[1]   S. Ahmedzai, 'Dying in Hospital: the Resident's Viewpoint', *British Medical Journal* 1982, 285, pp. 712–14.

[2] J. L. Cox, 'Care of the dying: Reflections of a Medical Student', *Canadian Medical Association Journal*, 136, 1987, pp. 577–9.

[3] A. Stedeford and R. G. Twycross, 'Care of the Patient With Advanced Cancer: a Course for Medical Students at Oxford, *Journal of Cancer Education* 4, 1989, pp. 103–8.

[4] F. M. Hull, 'Death, Dying and the Medical Student', *Medical Education* 25, 1991, pp. 491–6.

[5] B. M. Mount, personal communication.

*Further reading*

Brown, J. T. and Stoudemire, G. A., *Journal of the American Medical Association* 250, 1983, pp. 378–82.

Hinton, J., *Dying*, Penguin, Harmondsworth, 1967.

Kübler-Ross, E., *On Death and Dying*, Macmillan, New York, 1974.

Mount, B., Jones A. and Patterson, A., 'Death and Dying; Attitudes in a Teaching Hospital, *Urology* 4, 1974, pp. 27–33.

Osterweis, M., Solomon. F. and Green, M. (eds.), *Bereavement, Reactions, Consequence and Care*, National Academy Press, Washington, DC, 1984.

Parkes, C.M., *Bereavement*, Penguin, Harmondsworth, 1972.

Stroebe, W. and Stroebe, M. S., *Bereavement and Health*, Cambridge University Press, 1988.

# Chapter 12

*References*

[1] B. M Mount, personal communication.

[2] C. Buis, T. de Boo and R. Hull 'Touch and Breaking Bad News', *Family Practice* 8, 1991, pp. 303–4.

[3] R. Hull, 'Breaking Bad News' Videotape produced by Television Unit Police Headquarters, Leek Wootton, Warwickshire, England CV35 7QB, 1993.

*Further reading*

Autton, N., *Touch; an Exploration*, Darton, Longman and Todd, London, 1989.

Buckman, R. and Kason, Y., *How to Break Bad News*, Macmillan, London, 1992.

Hull, R., 'The Breast Lump in General Practice', in J. Coriel, R. Hull and V. J. Harten-Ash (eds.), *Current Approaches: Breaking Bad News*, Duphar Medical Relations, London, 1989.

Lichter, I., 'The Right to Bad News', in B. Stoll (ed.) *Ethical Dilemmas in Cancer Care*, Macmillan, Basingstoke, 1989.

Owens, R. G. and Naylor, F., *Living While Dying. What to Do and What to Say When You Are, or Someone Close to You Is Dying*, Thorsons, Wellingborough, 1989.

Appendix 1

# Helping agencies and support groups

## Introduction

Throughout the developed world there are many hundreds of national and regional organisations that offer help and support to people in need of palliative care. In a short book it is impossible to list them all. It would also be counterproductive because organisations and their addresses change. For this reason, only broad headings of helping agencies are listed with examples of each. In several countries directories of helping agencies are available in public libraries; they can supply up-to-date details of support groups and helping organisations.

*Australia*

See *Directory of Hospices and Palliative Care Services in Australia 1993*, South Australian Association for Hospice and Palliative Care (inc).

*Britain and Ireland*

*Directory of British Associations and Associations in Ireland*, Henderson G.P. and Henderson S.P.A. (eds), Kent CBD Research Ltd 1986

*Ireland*

*Administration Yearbook and Diary*, Institute of Public Administration, Dublin.

*Europe*

European Association for Palliative Care, National Cancer Institute of Milan, Via Venezian 1, 20133 Milan, Italy.

Centre de Soins Continus, I Chemin de la Savonniere, CH 1245 Collonge, Bellerive, Geneva, Switzerland.

*Canada*

The Canadian Palliative Care Association, 112, 43 rue Bruyere St, Ottawa, Ontario K1N 5C8.
(This association publishes a directory of services across the country.)

Directory of Associations, Micromedia.

*New Zealand*

See *Directory of Hospices and Palliative Care Services in New Zealand*, Hospice New Zealand, Wellington, PO Box 12481.

*United States*

*The Encyclopaedia of Associations*, Gruber, K. (ed.), Gale Research Company.

*World*

World Health Organization, Cancer and Palliative Care Unit, World Health Organization, 1211 Geneva 27, Switzerland.

## AIDS and HIV

*Britain*

AIDS Helpline, Tel. 0800 567 123.
Offers information and advice to any caller on all aspects of AIDS. A 24-hour, free, confidential service.

London Lighthouse, 111/117 Lancaster Rd, London W11 1QT, Tel. 01 792 1200.
AIDS hospice.

Terrence Higgins Trust, BM AIDS, London WC1N 3XX, Tel. 01 278 8745.

'Helpline' 01 833 2971 (7.00 pm–10.00 pm weekdays, 3.00 pm–10.00 pm weekends).

Provides information on AIDS and help and advice to sufferers and anyone worried about the disease.

At present there are no national organisations in North America but many urban centres have local advisory centres listed in local telephone directories.

## General cancer support groups

*Britain and Ireland*

BACUP (British Association of Cancer United Patients), 121/123 Charterhouse Street, London EC1M 6AA, Tel. 081 608 1661, 081 608 1785, 0800 181199 (freephone in UK).

Helps patients, their families and friends, cope with cancer. Trained cancer nurses provide information, emotional support and practical advice by telephone or letter. A range of free publications about colorectal and stomach cancer are available, together with fact sheets about cancer of the oesophagus and pancreas. A free newspaper is available. One-to-one counselling service in greater London area. 10.00 am–7.30 pm Mon–Thurs, 10.00 am–5 pm Fridays.

Cancer Link, 17 Britannia Street, London WC1 9JN, Tel. 071 833 2451 Scotland. Tel. 031 228 5557.

Information and emotional support, telephone or letter enquiries on all aspects of cancer, from people with cancer, families, friends and professionals.
Resource to over 300 cancer support and self-help groups in the UK. Free publications on request.

The Malcolm Sargent Cancer Fund for Children, 14 Abingdon Road, London W8 6AF, Tel. 081 937 4548.

Can provide cash grants for parents of children up to the age of 21 with cancer, to help pay for clothing, equipment, travel, fuel bills, etc. Apply through the hospital social worker, who will fill in a form on the patient's behalf.

Marie Curie Cancer Care, 28 Belgrave Square, London SW1X 8QG, Tel. 081 235 3325.

Nursing care available in eleven Marie Curie homes in the UK. Admission details through individual matrons. Day/night nursing provided in patient's home through community nursing services, administered through local health authority. Welfare grant schemes through district nursing services.

Irish Cancer Society, Information Officer, 5 Northumberland Road, Dublin 4, Republic of Ireland, Tel. 0001 681855 or dial 10 and ask for 'Freefone Cancer' (*Ireland only*).

Information on all aspects of cancer from nurses via freefone service. Funds home care and rehabilitation programmes run by voluntary groups, for all cancer patients. Support groups for mastectomy, colostomy and laryngectomy patients, Hodgkins disease advice. Home night nursing services available on request of patient's doctor or public health nurse. Publishes: 'What you should know about Cancer' which discusses various risk factors that predispose to gastrointestinal cancer.

The Ulster Cancer Foundation, 40–42 Eglantine Avenue, Belfast, BT9 6DX Northern Ireland, Tel. 0232 663281/2/3. Helpline: 0232 663439 (9.30 am–12.30 pm weekdays).

Involved in many aspects of cancer, from prevention to patient support. Operates an information helpline for cancer-related queries for patients and their families, staffed by experienced cancer nurses, who can arrange counselling by personal appointment at the centre.

Rehabilitation support services include; mastectomy advice (volunteer visiting by former patients) laryngectomy clubs (monthly activities, support in hospitals and at home), lymphoma support (patient and family link-up).

*Australia*

Australian Cancer Society Inc., GPO Box 4708, Sydney 2001, Tel. (02) 358 2066.

There are cancer support services in each Australian state as follows:

- ACT: PO Box 316, Curtin 2605, Tel. (06) 285 3070.
- NSW: PO Box 572, Kings Cross 2011,
  Tel. (02) 334 1900.
- NT: PO Box 42719, Casuarina 0811,
  Tel. (089) 27 4888.
- Qld: PO Box 201, Spring Hill 4004,
  Tel. (07) 257 1155.
- SA: PO Box 160, North Adelaide 5006,
  Tel. (08) 267 5222.
- Tas. South: 13 Liverpool St, Hobart 7000,
  Tel. (002) 31 2990.
- Tas. North: PO Box 475, Launceston 7250,
  Tel. (003) 31 6433.
- Vic.: Rathdowne St, Carlton South 3053,
  Tel. (03) 279 1111.
- WA: 334 Rokeby Rd, Subiaco 6008,
  Tel. (09) 381 4515.

*United States and Canada*

American Cancer Society, 90 Park Avenue, New York, New York 10016, Tel. (212) 599–3600.

Exceptional Cancer Patients Inc., 2 Church Street S, New Haven, CT 06519, Tel. (203) 865–8392.

Offers help to patients searching for information on how to live with the disease, reduce stress and resolve conflicts; including tapes and videos.

The International Association of Cancer Victors and Friends Inc., 7740 W. Manchester Ave, Ste. 110, Playa del Rey, CA 90293, Tel. (213) 822–5032.

This non-profitmaking organisation offers educational information on little known non-toxic alternative therapies. It also has groups in Australia and Canada.

Make Today Count, Box 222, Osage Beach, MO 65065, Tel. (314) 348–1619.

Canadian Cancer Society, 77 Bloor Street W., Ste. 1702, Toronto, Ontario M5S 3A1, Tel. (416) 961–7223.

## Breast cancer support groups

*Britain*

Breast Care & Mastectomy Association of Great Britain, 26a Harrison Street, Kings Cross, London WC1 8JG, Tel. 071 837 0908.

Personal callers, by appointment. Volunteers throughout UK (all have had breast surgery). Offers home visits on a local basis. Offers support on a one-to-one basis to women who have had, or are about to have breast surgery. Prostheses for partial or whole breast loss, AAA–DD sizes. Books & leaflets free to individuals.
Cassette tape £2.00, video cassette £29.90 (inc.VAT) plus £2.00 pp.
Run 1 day seminars for health professionals 10–3.30 (details on request, SAE).

*Canada*

Alliance of Breast Cancer Survivors, 20 Eglinton Avenue West, Suite 1106, Toronto, Ontario M4R 1K8, Tel. (416) 487–9899.

## Colostomy support groups

*Britain and Ireland*

British Colostomy Association, 38–39 Eccleston Square, London SW1V 1PB, Tel. 071 828 5175.

Information and advisory service. Giving comfort, reassurance and encouragement to return to previous lifestyle. Personal and confidential emotional support by helpers who have experience of living with a colostomy. Free leaflets and lists of local contacts. Publishes booklets about colostomy care in many languages. Can arrange visits to hospital or home on request.

Ileostomy Association of Great Britain & Ireland, Amblehurst House, Black Scotch Lane, Mansfield, NG18 4PF, Tel. 0623 28 099.

The association offers a wide range of advisory services through local committee members as well as national advisors. It also publishes *The Ileostomy Book*.

Worldwide International Ostomy Association, c/o British Colostomy Association, 38/39 Eccleston Square, London SW1V 1PB, Tel. 071 828 5175.

The IOA is an international organisation based in the USA, which publishes the *Ostomy International Magazine*.

*United States*

United Ostomy Association, 36 Executive Park, Suite 120, Irvine, California, USA 92714.

## Eye cancer support groups

Blindness, British Council for Prevention of, 12 Harcourt St, London W1H 1DS, Tel. 081 724 3716.

Blind Society (Jewish), 221 Golders Green Rd, London NW11, Tel. 081 458 3282.

Glaucoma Association (International), Kings College Hospital, Denmark Hill, London SE5 9RS, Tel. 081 274 6222 ext 2453.

Royal National Institute for the Blind, Braille House, 338–346 Grosswell Road, London, ECIV 7SE.

*United States and Canada*

American Foundation for the Blind, 15 West 16th St, New York, New York 10011, Tel. (212) 620–2000.

Canadian National Institute for the Blind, 1929 Bayview Avenue, Toronto, Ontario M4W 3P2, Tel. (416) 486–2500.

# Head and neck cancer support groups

*Britain*

Let's face it, 10 Woodend, Crowthorne, Berks RG11 6DQ, Tel. 0344 774405.

Contact point for people of any age coping with facial disfigurement. Provides a link for people with similar experiences.

*Canada*

Look Good ... Feel Better, Canadian Cosmetic, Toiletry and Fragrance Association Foundation, 5090 Explorer Drive, Suite 510, Mississauga, Ontario L4W 4T9.

# Hodgkins disease support groups

*Britain*

Hodgkin's Disease Association, PO Box 275 Haddenham, Aylesbury, Bucks HP17 8JJ, Tel. 0844 291500.

Provides information and emotional support for lymphoma patients and their families. Literature and video available. National network of helpers with experience of the disease, enquirers usually linked by telephone.

# Hospice information

*Britain*

Hospice Information Service, 51/53 Lawrie Park Road, Sydenham SE26 6DZ.

Can provide further information about location of nearest hospice and the facilities provided.

*Australia*

Australian states are represented in the Australian Association for Hospice and Palliative Care Inc. Addresses for each state are:

- ACT: PO Box 88, Civic Square 2608, Tel. (06) 253 1053.

- NSW: c/o Calvary Hospital, PO Box 261, Kogarah 2217, Tel. (02) 587 8333.

- Qld: PO Box 63, Woolloongabba 4102, Tel. (07) 240 1111.

- SA: PO Box 275, Belair 5052, Tel. (08) 278 7402.

- Tas.: PO Box 136, Lindisfarne 7015, Tel. (002) 43 9480.

- Vic.: PO Box 1200, North Fitzroy 3068, Tel. (03) 486 2666.

- WA: Health Yourself House, 334 Rokeby Rd, Subiaco 6008, Tel. (09) 381 4515.

- NT: PO Box 42255, Casuarina 0811, Tel. (089) 27 4888.

# Hysterectomy support groups

*Britain*

Hysterectomy Support, c/o WHRIC, 52 Featherstone St, London EC1 8RT, Tel. 081 251 6332/6580 (11.00 am–5.00 pm Mon., Wed., Fri).

Refers women, family or partners, concerned about hysterectomy, to former patients in their areas. Provides encouragement, advice and support, through informal sharing of information and experiences.

## Laryngectomy support groups
*Britain*
> National Association of Laryngectomy Clubs, 4th floor, 39 Eccleston Square, London SW1V 1PB, Tel. 081 834 2857.

Promotes the welfare of laryngectomies within the UK. Encourages the formation of clubs with objectives of assisting rehabilitation through speech therapy, social support and monthly meetings. Advises on speech aids and medical supplies.

*United States*
> International Association of Laryngectomies, 1599 Clifton Road NE, Atlanta, Georgia USA 30329.

## Leukaemia support groups
*Britain*
> Leukaemia Care Society, PO Box 82 Exeter, Devon EX2 5DP, Tel. 0392 218514.

Promotes the welfare of people with leukaemia and allied blood disorders.
Offers family caravan holidays, friendship and support via volunteer area secretaries throughout UK.

## Pelvic support groups
*Britain*
> Pelvic Exenteration Group (PEG), 35 Dunton Road, Kingshurst B37 6JH, Tel. 788 2161.

Offers information services, support groups, welfare rights, where to obtain underwear/swimwear.

## Urostomy support groups
*Britain*
> Urostomy Association, Buckland, Beaumont Park, Danbury, Essex CM3 4DE, Tel. 024 541 4294.

Assists patients before and after surgery, with counselling on appliances, housing, work situations or marital problems. Helps them to resume as full a life as possible with confidence.

## Bereavement support groups
> Cruse Bereavement Care, Cruse House, 126 Sheen Road, Richmond, Surrey, Tel. 081 940 4818.

Offers individual and group bereavement, by trained counsellors. Advice and information on practical problems and social contact.

## Carers support groups
*Britain*
> Counselling Help and Advice Together (CHAT), 20 Cavendish Square, London W1M 0AB, Tel. 071 629 3870 or 071 409 3333.

Personal and individual service. Counsellors and advisers offer counselling, help and information on a range of problems including: personal matters, stress, pre-retirement/retirement, rehabilitation, illness, bereavement, distress.

## Parents support groups
*Britain*
> The Compassionate Friend, 6 Denmark Street, Bristol BSI 5DQ, Tel. 0272 292778.

Self-help group of parents who have lost a son or daughter of any age including adult. Quarterly newsletter, postal library, range of leaflets, personal and group support, befriending rather than counselling.

> The Malcolm Sargent Cancer Fund for Children, 14 Abingdon Road London W8 6AF, Tel. 081 937 4548.

Can provide cash grants for parents of children up to the age of 21 with cancer, to help pay for clothing, equipment, travel, fuel bills etc. Apply through a hospital Social Worker in Britain.

> National Advisory Service for Parents of Children with a Stoma, (NASPCS), 32 Suters Drive, Thorpe Marriott, Taverham, Norwich, Norfolk NR8 6UU, Tel. 0603 860373.

The service is for all children with a stoma or who are incontinent. It provides a contact service that gives moral support and practical advice.
It publishes a quarterly newsletter and *Our Special Children*, which is a practical guide to stoma care in babies and young children.

> Society of Parents of Children with Cancer, Parent Contact Service, 7 Holebank Road, Hall Green, Birmingham B28 8EU, Tel. 778 2538.

Offers self-help support groups for parents/children, social functions.
Holiday camp on Welsh/English border. Other holidays for SPOCC children.
Redirects to other organisations for 'dreams come true'.

*United States and Canada*
> Candlelighter Childhood Cancer Foundation, 2025 Eye St, NW, Ste. 1011, Washington DC 20006. Tel. (202) 659–5136.

Candlelighter Childhood Cancer Foundation Canada, 10 Alcorn Avenue, Suite 200, Toronto, Ontario M2P 1H4.

Offers parent support groups in the US and Canada for families of children with cancer.

# Hydromorphone

Hydromorphone, a semi-synthetic pure opioid agonist, is a hydrogenated ketone of morphine, shares the pharmacologic properties of typical opiate analgesics and is about five times more potent than morphine. Though not available in Britain it has been used to treat cancer pain in North America since 1932.

Onset of pain control is rapid (occurring within 10–15 minutes) by oral and parenteral routes, but delayed when taken rectally. Side-effects are minimal; some patients who cannot tolerate nausea and anorexia with morphine experience no similar problem with hydromorphone. Only a few cases of drowsiness develop and hydromorphone causes less constipation than morphine.

Respiratory depression has been observed more frequently with hydromorphone than with morphine. Withdrawal reactions are milder than with morphine. Hydromorphone suppositories are more rapid in action and have a longer duration than other opioid suppositories. Hydromorphone is available as Dilaudid in 1, 2, 3, and 4 mg tablets and injections and as 3 mg suppositories.

Hydromorphone is an effective narcotic for the treatment of cancer pain. Many authorities recommend hydromorphone as a first-line narcotic with an analgesic efficacy similar to morphine. Hydromorphone achieves its equivalent analgesic action at a dosage approximately 15–20% of that of morphine. Hydromorphone may be particularly useful for patients who develop a tolerance to morphine, who suffer from debilitating side-effects of morphine or who require parenteral therapy for pain control using small volumes of fluids.

The increasing use of hydromorphone in Canada for cancer and other forms of moderate to severe pain appears to have resulted from the recent availability of a high potency parenteral formulation (Dilaudid HP) and its recognised effectiveness as a narcotic.

Complete control of pain in cancer patients is now considered to be possible in most cases. Hydromorphone represents an efficacious and well-tolerated narcotic to help to achieve this goal. Its advantages make it a valuable alternative to morphine.

# Index